Stem Cells

by Peggy J. Parks

Current Issues

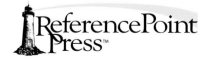
ReferencePoint Press™

San Diego, CA

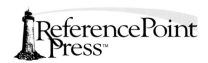

© 2009 ReferencePoint Press, Inc.

For more information, contact:
ReferencePoint Press, Inc.
PO Box 27779
San Diego, CA 92198
www.ReferencePointPress.com

Picture credits:
Maury Aaseng: 32–35, 48–51, 64–67, 81–83
Landov: 11, 15

Parks, Peggy J., 1951–
  Stem cells / by Peggy J. Parks.
      p. cm. —(Compact research series)
  Includes bibliographical references and index.
  ISBN-13: 978-1-60152-051-7 (hardback)
  ISBN-10: 1-60152-051-4 (hardback)
  1. Stem cells. I. Title.
  QH588.S83.P368 2008
  616'.02774—dc22   2008008810

Contents

Foreword

As modern civilization continues to evolve, its ability to create, store, distribute, and access information expands exponentially. The explosion of information from all media continues to increase at a phenomenal rate. By 2020 some experts predict the worldwide information base will double every 73 days. While access to diverse sources of information and perspectives is paramount to any democratic society, information alone cannot help people gain knowledge and understanding. Information must be organized and presented clearly and succinctly in order to be understood. The challenge in the digital age becomes not the creation of information, but how best to sort, organize, enhance, and present information.

ReferencePoint Press developed the *Compact Research* series with this challenge of the information age in mind. More than any other subject area today, researching current issues can yield vast, diverse, and unqualified information that can be intimidating and overwhelming for even the most advanced and motivated researcher. The *Compact Research* series offers a compact, relevant, intelligent, and conveniently organized collection of information covering a variety of current topics ranging from illegal immigration and methamphetamine to diseases such as anorexia and meningitis.

The series focuses on three types of information: objective single-author narratives, opinion-based primary source quotations, and facts and statistics. The clearly written objective narratives provide context and reliable background information. Primary source quotes are carefully selected and cited, exposing the reader to differing points of view. And facts and statistics sections aid the reader in evaluating perspectives. Presenting these key types of information creates a richer, more balanced learning experience.

For better understanding and convenience, the series enhances information by organizing it into narrower topics and adding design features that make it easy for a reader to identify desired content. For example, in *Compact Research: Illegal Immigration*, a chapter covering the economic impact of illegal immigration has an objective narrative explaining the various ways the economy is impacted, a balanced section of numerous primary source quotes on the topic, followed by facts and full-color illustrations to encourage evaluation of contrasting perspectives.

The ancient Roman philosopher Lucius Annaeus Seneca wrote, "It is quality rather than quantity that matters." More than just a collection of content, the *Compact Research* series is simply committed to creating, finding, organizing, and presenting the most relevant and appropriate amount of information on a current topic in a user-friendly style that invites, intrigues, and fosters understanding.

Stem Cells at a Glance

The Importance of Stem Cells

Although living things are made up of trillions of cells, stem cells are unique because they are the parent cells, with the ability to create all the different cells in the body.

Types of Stem Cells

The stem cells in an embryo are known as embryonic stem cells. As these stem cells mature they become adult stem cells, which are specialized to different parts of the body. If stem cells are isolated and grown in culture, they form families known as stem cell lines.

Where Are Stem Cells Found?

A three- to five-day-old embryo (known as a blastocyst) contains embryonic stem cells. Adult stem cells are found throughout the tissues and organs of developed humans, and are also found in placenta and umbilical cord blood. Recent research has shown that stem cells found in amniotic fluid have characteristics much like embryonic stem cells. Somatic cell nuclear transfer (SCNT) is used to create cloned embryos, but scientists have not yet succeeded in extracting stem cells from them.

Medical Progress and Potential

Adult stem cells from bone marrow and umbilical blood are used to treat numerous diseases and conditions. Although embryonic stem cells are not yet used in any human treatments, researchers are hopeful that they will eventually be used to develop treatments and cures for Parkinson's and Alzheimer's disease, as well as other diseases.

Risks

Embryonic stem cells have been shown to develop teratomas, or "monster tumors," in research animals. Another potential risk with embryonic stem cells is that if they are injected into humans, they could be recognized as foreign by the body's immune system and rejected or destroyed. Known risks of adult stem cell treatments include infection, tissue rejection, and graft versus host disease (GVHD).

Ethical Issues

The greatest controversy is over embryonic stem cell research because it involves destroying human embryos in order to remove their stem cells, which some people believe is the same as killing a human being. The cloning of embryos is also an issue of controversy.

Stem Cell Research Regulation

In the United States, the Food and Drug Administration (FDA) tightly regulates scientific research, including that which involves stem cells. All new medical procedures, drugs, and treatments must go through rigorous, time-consuming animal tests and human trials before they can be released to the public. Currently, the FDA directs what diseases can be treated by bone marrow and umbilical cord stem cells, and forbids the use of embryonic stem cells for human treatments.

Overview

❝Stem cells are like little kids who, when they grow up, can enter a variety of professions. A child might become a fireman, a doctor or a plumber, depending on the influences in their life—or environment. In the same way, these stem cells can become many tissues by making certain changes in their environment.❞

—Marc Hedrick, quoted in UCLA news release, "UCLA/Pitt Researchers Transform Human Fat into Bone, Muscle, Cartilage."

❝Without stem cells, wounds would never heal, your skin and blood could not continually renew themselves, fertilized eggs would not grow into babies, and babies would not grow into adults.❞

—*Nature*, "What Are Stem Cells?"

For centuries scientists have known that living organisms are made up of cells, which are the basic building blocks of life. The bodies of humans and other mammals contain trillions of cells of more than 200 different types, from red and white blood cells to neurons, or cells of the nervous system. But among this massive collection of cells, some have qualities that set them apart from others. These are known as stem cells, the master cells of the body from which all other cells are created.

Stem cells are found throughout the body's tissues and organs at all stages of life, before and after birth. The reason they are so unique is that unlike ordinary cells, which have a specialized purpose such as carrying oxygen through the blood or fighting infection, stem cells are unspecialized, or "programmable." They have the miraculous ability to take on the characteristics of different cells in tissues and organs, a process known as differentiation. Scientist Christopher Thomas Scott writes: "Every passing hour represents a turning point for a stem cell, and the trajectory of change is overwhelmingly in one direction: cells are destined to become specialists in a fully functioning organism."[1] Another reason stem cells are unique is that they can renew themselves indefinitely through constant cell division. When stem cells divide, daughter cells form; one daughter cell acts as the parent, keeping the stem cell characteristics and remaining behind to continue dividing. The offspring, known as a progenitor cell, moves on to differentiate and form cells with more specialized, organ-specific functions.

"The Ultimate Stem Cell"

Embryonic stem cells come from an embryo, a term that refers to the various stages of development beginning with fertilization of an egg by sperm. Once an egg has been fertilized, the two cells fuse together to form a single cell, the earliest form of an embryo known as a zygote. At this point the embryo is totipotent, meaning it has the capability to generate all the different cells necessary to form a complete organism. As *Nature Reports* explains: "A fertilized egg is the ultimate stem cell, as it is the source of every type of cell in the body, from oxygen-carrying red blood cells to electricity-conducting nerve cells and throbbing heart muscle cells."[2] The zygote splits into two cells, then four, then eight, and as it keeps dividing the cells get smaller and smaller. When the embryo is between four and six days old it has become a fluid-filled ball called a blastocyst, which is so tiny it could fit on the head of a pin. The blastocyst is composed of an outer layer of cells and an inner cell mass, which is the source of embryonic stem cells. If it is implanted in a woman's womb, the outer layer of cells eventually forms the placenta and amniotic tissue, and the inner cell mass develops

> " Stem cells are found throughout the body's tissues and organs at all stages of life, before and after birth. "

into all the tissues that make up the fetus's body.

If, however, the stem cells are extracted from the embryo and grown in vitro, or a controlled, artificial environment such as a petri dish, they continue to divide and multiply indefinitely, forming families of cells known as stem cell lines. These stem cells are pluripotent, which means they are capable of changing into every type of cell in the body with the exception of placenta. Most human embryonic stem cells are generated from embryos created through in vitro fertilization for couples who are unable to conceive naturally. To maximize the chances of a successful pregnancy, the mother takes fertility drugs so she will produce multiple eggs. Then the eggs are extracted and fertilized in test tubes. If more than one egg becomes fertile and spare embryos result, the parents have several options. They may have the fertility clinic freeze the spare embryos for possible future pregnancies, give them up for adoption by other parents, or direct that they be destroyed. In some countries, including the United States, parents can donate the spare embryos for research.

> " Because adult stem cells are found in the tissues of all humans from babies to adults, their more accurate name is somatic stem cells, meaning 'of the body.' "

Adult Stem Cells

As embryonic stem cells continue to mature, they eventually become adult stem cells. Adult stem cells are multipotent, or capable of producing a limited number of cell types. Once they commit to a pathway of differentiation, they become more and more specialized to the tissue where they eventually reside. Pulitzer prize–winning science journalist Gareth Cook explains:

> Scientists believe that the cells of the body form a kind of family tree, with the embryonic stem cell at the trunk and most of the multitude of cells that make up the body

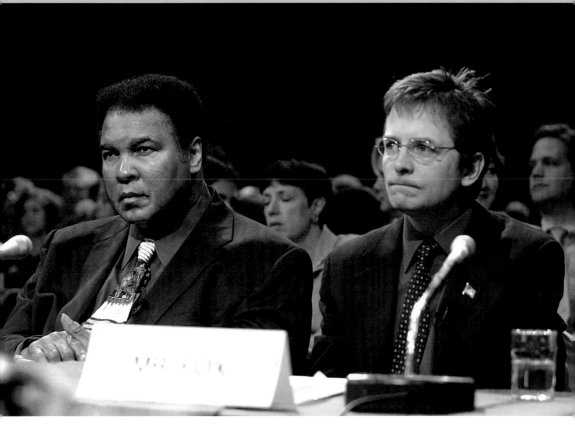

Michael J. Fox, (right) attending a Senate Appropriations Subcommittee with former boxer Muhammad Ali (left), is a well-known actor and advocate of all types of stem cell research. Both men suffer from Parkinson's disease and encourage Congress to increase funding and support for stem cell research.

at the tips of the branches. . . . [A]s the embryo develops, different cells start to travel down different branches in the family of cells, becoming more specialized and less flexible, in a process called commitment. Stem cells that are partway down one of these branches are called adult stem cells because they are destined to become specific types of tissue in the adult and are thought to have lost the full potential of embryonic stem cells."[3]

Some adult stem cells are capable of making several different cell types, while others, including those found in skin, intestines, and blood, are limited to producing only one kind of specialized cell.

Because adult stem cells are found in the tissues of all humans from babies to adults, their more accurate name is somatic stem cells, meaning "of the body." Numerous organs and tissues contain adult stem cells, including the heart, brain, skeletal muscle, skin, liver, lymph nodes, circulating blood and blood vessels, as well as umbilical cord and placenta. A particularly rich source of adult stem cells is bone marrow, the soft, spongy tissue inside bone cavities that produces white blood cells, red blood cells, and tiny blood-clotting cells known as platelets. It is widely believed that adult stem cells live in their own specific areas of tissue and remain quiescent (nondividing) until they are activated by injury or disease; then they spring into action and form new cells to heal damaged tissue. In this way, adult stem cells serve as a built-in repair kit for the body.

Cloned Stem Cells

In recent years many scientists have focused their stem cell research on somatic cell nuclear transfer (SCNT), or cloning. In this procedure, an egg is surgically removed from a woman's body, and the nucleus, which contains her unique genetic information (DNA), is removed from the egg. Then a body cell, often from skin or muscle, is taken from someone else (either male or female), and its DNA is removed from the cell and inserted into the "empty" egg. After a zap of electrical current, the egg is tricked into behaving as though it has been fertilized, and it begins to divide and grow like a normal embryo. Theoretically, once a cloned embryo has been created, its stem cells could be removed and grown into cloned stem cell lines. To date, however, this exists only in theory; no scientist has ever been able to achieve it.

In June 2005 it appeared that South Korean researcher Hwang Woo-suk had finally achieved what no other scientist had been able to do. Hwang was lauded worldwide as a scientific pioneer after reportedly creating 11 lines of human embryonic stem cells from cloned embryos—but his claims turned out to be fraudulent. A panel of experts appointed to investigate his research found that all the allegedly cloned stem cell lines were fakes. Hwang later apologized, but his deceit stunned the scientific world; Donald Kennedy, editor in chief of *Science* magazine, refers to it as "one of the most comprehensive and convincing frauds in the history of research misconduct."[4]

Even though no stem cell lines have been created from cloned embryos, scientists throughout the United States and other countries are aggressively pursuing SCNT research. In January 2008 scientists at the California firm Stemagen Corporation said that they had created cloned embryos using ordinary skin cells, but they were not able to produce any stem cells. According to researcher George Daley of the Harvard Institute and Children's Hospital Boston, SCNT research is progressing well, and it will not be long before cloned stem cells are created. "The real holy grail is to generate a pluripotent stem cell line from a cloned human blastocyst," he says. "It's only a matter of time before some group succeeds."[5]

Is Stem Cell Research Necessary?

Stem cell research is often hailed by scientists as the most promising hope for the future of medicine. Because stem cells are so versatile and have such unique properties, researchers have long been excited about how they might be used in developing treatments and cures for disease and debilitating injuries. California's Steenblock Research Institute is particularly exuberant in its description of stem cells, calling them "mysterious, magical, life altering, life enhancing, life prolonging, life saving, wonder cells!"[6]

Embryonic stem cell research is a young field that is still in the animal-testing stage, but adult stem cell treatments have achieved medical progress for many years. In the past, people who were diagnosed with leukemia, immune deficiency diseases, or hereditary blood disorders, were often given little hope for survival. Now, because of stem cell transplants from bone marrow and umbilical cord blood, many children and adults have been cured and are living normal, healthy lives.

Which Stem Cells Are the Most Promising?

Even though embryonic stem cell research is still in its infancy, many scientists are convinced that its potential is superior to that of adult stem cells. Adult stem cells are mature and specialized, so they are not as versatile as embryonic stem cells. *Nature Reports* explains: "Tissue-specific stem cells appear to be specialists, quite good at making a few types of cells. Stem cells found in bone marrow naturally make new red blood cells and new white blood cells, for instance, but not new brain cells."[7] Another way researchers explain this is that adult stem cells have less plasticity than embryonic stem cells. Also, adult stem cells are hidden deep within tissues, exist in very low numbers, and are surrounded by millions of ordinary cells. As a result, adult stem cells are rare and difficult for scientists to locate and identify. Even when these cells have been isolated and are grown in culture, they grow very, very slowly. This makes it extremely difficult for researchers to produce enough of the cells to be therapeutically useful.

> "Stem cell research is often hailed by scientists as the most promising hope for the future of medicine."

Embryonic stem cells, however, multiply and grow rapidly as well as indefinitely. They are easier for scientists to collect, purify, and maintain in culture than are adult stem cells. And they retain their stem cell characteristics, along with their capacity to produce the more than 200 cell types that are found throughout the body. Scientists have developed methods of turning embryonic stem cells into brain, heart, and muscle cells, as well as blood cells, blood vessel cells, and bone cells, and they believe the potential is virtually unlimited. According to renowned stem cell researcher Irving Weissman, it is clear that embryonic stem cells have far more potential than adult stem cells. He explains:

> Several opponents [of embryonic stem cell research] previously have claimed that any adult stem cell could turn into any other tissue, and so neither embryonic stem cell research nor nuclear transfer stem cell research would be necessary. Although this notion has been thoroughly disproven by several independent groups, those advocates persist in their claims. While we can hope that such disinformation is not accepted by the public, I fear that these claims are now being viewed through the lenses of politics and of the media, and not on the basis of medical or scientific evidence.[8]

Is Stem Cell Research Ethical?

Various ethical concerns have been raised about stem cell research, including SCNT cloning. Although it is intended strictly for research

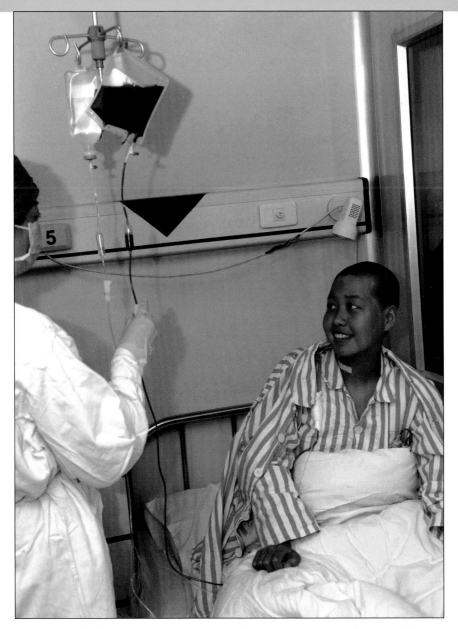

This young leukemia patient receives a bone marrow transplant in China. Donated stem cells are being used in her treatment.

or for possible therapeutic uses, it essentially involves the same process that is used to clone animals. Human reproductive cloning is denounced among scientists as being deplorable and unethical, but some people still fear that unscrupulous researchers will eventually use SCNT to clone human beings. This is the perspective of Wesley J. Smith, who is a senior fellow at the Discovery Institute and a special consultant for the Center for Bioethics and Culture. He writes: "The same procedure used to create a cloned human embryo for research could also be used to bring about the birth of the first cloned baby. Indeed, attempts are already underway to make this dreaded prospect a reality."[9]

As controversial as SCNT is, the most hotly debated aspect of stem cell research is the destruction of human embryos for the purpose of extracting their stem cells. Those who strongly object to human embryonic stem cell research believe human life begins at conception—that as tiny and undeveloped as embryos are, they are unquestionably human, as James Sherley, associate professor of biological engineering at the Massachusetts Institute of Technology (MIT), explains: "What else could they be—aliens? Scientists who want to conduct experiments with human embryos are quick to say what human embryos are not. I challenge them to tell the public what human embryos are. There is only one answer to this question, 'living human beings.'"[10] Opponents of human embryonic stem cell research often equate embryo destruction with abortion, pointing out that many leftover embryos have been adopted and have grown into healthy children. Destroying them to benefit science, they say, is morally and ethically wrong.

> "The most hotly debated aspect of stem cell research is the destruction of human embryos for the purpose of extracting their stem cells.

Supporters of embryonic stem cell research acknowledge that an embryo has the potential to become a human, but they say it is not the same as a living, breathing human being. They often point out that most leftover embryos at fertility clinics are destroyed anyway and could be put to good use for stem cell research. Actor Michael J. Fox, who suffers from Parkinson's disease, is an outspoken advocate of embryonic stem cell research. His Michael J. Fox Foundation is dedicated to finding a cure for Parkinson's, as well as ensuring the development of improved therapies designed to help people who are living with the disease. Another supporter, Michael Kinsley, is a political journalist suffering from Parkinson's disease. He explains: "The embryos used in stem-cell research come from fertility clinics, which would otherwise discard them. . . . Why let these embryos go to waste?"[11]

A Tremendous Scientific Milestone

As scientists pursue stem cell research, they continue to make exciting progress. One of the most promising discoveries in stem cell research was announced in November 2007. Working independently from each other in different parts of the world, researchers James A. Thomson of the United States and Shinya Yamanaka of Japan successfully reprogrammed normal human skin cells to become stem cells with all the versatility and pluripotency of embryonic stem cells. Although the research is preliminary, it has been hailed by scientists throughout the world as a major breakthrough. Robert Lanza, chief science officer of Advanced Technology, explains why this is such an important accomplishment: "To be able to take a few cells from a patient—say a cheek swab or a few skin cells—and turn them into stem cells in the laboratory. . . . This work represents a tremendous scientific milestone—the biological equivalent of the Wright Brothers' first airplane. It's a bit like learning how to turn lead into gold."[12]

Are Stem Cells the Answer to Prolonged Human Life?

Even though scientists have diverse opinions about which type of stem cell research should be pursued, most overwhelmingly agree that it has incomparable potential to allow humans to live longer, healthier lives. Researchers are optimistic that stem cells will lead to cures for many diseases and disorders, including Parkinson's disease, Alzheimer's disease, and multiple sclerosis, as well as treatments for severe burns and spinal cord injuries. In experiments with rats, professor Hans Kierstead used embryonic stem cells to cure damaged spinal cords. Before the treatment, one of the rats was unable to walk normally; instead, its hindquarters dragged along the floor of the cage as it feebly attempted to move, with its tail trailing limply behind. Kierstead differentiated embryonic stem cells into neural cells and then injected them into the rat seven days after its spinal cord was injured. Within two months the rat had regained its ability to walk with only the slightest suggestion of a limp.

Researchers from the Massachusetts Institute of Technology made a discovery with stem cells that could potentially save millions of lives. Mice were genetically altered to have sickle-cell anemia, a hereditary disease of the bone marrow that is often fatal. The researchers took cells from the skin of the diseased mice and reprogrammed them to become embryonic-like stem cells. Then they differentiated the stem cells to become precursors of bone marrow adult stem cells and injected them back into the mice. Afterward, tests showed that the creatures' blood and kidney functions were normal and that all symptoms of their disease had vanished. Scientists are hopeful that this research will eventually lead to a cure for sickle-cell anemia.

Potential Risks of Stem Cell Treatment

Throughout the history of medicine, every new vaccination, drug, treatment, and procedure has carried a certain amount of risk, and stem cells are no exception. Some researchers say that the greatest risk is with embryonic stem cells. One reason is their potential for rejection: If embryonic stem cells are implanted in humans, the immune systems would recognize the cells as foreign and likely reject or destroy them, in the same way that organs may be rejected after organ transplants. An even greater risk that has been identified in numerous animal studies is that when the creatures are injected with embryonic stem cells they develop bizarre tumors known as teratomas, or "monster tumors," that contain bits of teeth, bone, and muscle, as well as primitive eyes and tufts of hair. Although teratomas are benign rather than cancerous, if they grow too large they can be deadly. Several studies have shown that from 70 to 100 percent of experimental animals died as a result of teratomas. As researcher Maureen L. Condic explains: "When cells derived from embryonic stem cells are transplanted into adult animals, their most common fate is to die."[13]

Although adult stem cell therapy is generally accepted as the safer approach, it, too, carries potential risks, such as tissue rejection and infection. A rare but potentially fatal risk is graft versus host disease, or GVHD, which can result if immune system cells from a donor inadvertently make their way into the patient's bloodstream. GVHD is most common following bone marrow transplants and can lead to a variety of complications ranging from nausea and cramping to bloody diarrhea and death. GVHD is divided into two categories: acute, which affects the skin, gastrointestinal tract, and liver; and chronic, which affects nearly every organ in the body. According to journalist Steven Edwards, the National Center for Health Statistics reports that between 2000 and 2004, adult stem cells used in 25,000 bone marrow transplants in the United States resulted in 3,629 deaths, of which 624 were children under the age of 18.

Adult stem cells have also been connected with cancer. A team of scientists in Madrid, Spain, extracted adult stem cells from fat tissue, grew them in culture, and then transplanted them into animals. The oldest of the stem cells formed cancers, leading some researchers to conclude that when adult stem cells replicate too many times, they can become cancerous. If that is correct, it means that adult stem cells stored for too long may not be safe for human use.

Can the Stem Cell Debate Be Resolved?

Of all the issues related to science and research, stem cells are among the most emotion-charged, highly publicized, and political. In 2001 George W. Bush became the first U.S. president to approve federal funding for embryonic stem cell research. He stipulated, however, that the money could be used only for existing lines from embryos that had already been destroyed, not for the stem cells derived through the destruction of new embryos. In 2006 and 2007 Bush vetoed proposed legislation that would have expanded funding for embryonic stem cell research, saying that he would not support federal monies being used for the deliberate destruction of human embryos. Although he has been criticized for his stance on embryonic stem cell research, many people share his viewpoint. William Hurlbut, who is a consulting professor of neuroscience at Stanford University, shares his perspective: "A great many people object to this. It's not just religious people. The truth is that the country is very deeply divided."[14] Because of the restrictions on federal funding, most embryonic stem cell research is financed through private grants and donations.

As researchers continue to explore new options and make breakthrough discoveries, the day may eventually come when the controversy ends and stem cells live up to their potential for vastly improving human health. Yet no one can say when—or even if—the stem cell debate will ever truly be resolved.

Is Stem Cell Research Necessary?

66 Stem cell research . . . is considered by the world's brightest scientific minds to be a true revolution in the way we view and treat disease. 99

—Eve Herold, *Stem Cell Wars: Inside Stories from the Frontlines.*

66 As with many other contemporary debates in biology and biotechnology, the stem cell controversy is hard to escape, yet is too often characterized by hype and confusion. 99

—Council for Responsible Genetics (CRG), "What Your Mother Never Told You About Stem Cells."

Despite the controversies over stem cell research, most scientists agree that it is absolutely crucial and must continue to move forward. Studies and experiments with adult stem cells have produced cures for diseases that were once thought to be untreatable, and certainly incurable. Through research with embryonic and cloned stem cells, scientists are hopeful that even more cures and treatments will be possible in the coming years. John Kessler, neurology professor and chairman of the Department of Neurology at Northwestern University's Feinberg School of Medicine, explains why scientists are so excited about stem cell research: "It's quite breathtaking when you think about all the ways in which stem cells can affect medicine. All those horrible diseases that we can't treat right now will be able to be treated in the future."[15]

Scientific Firsts

Researchers theorized about the existence of unique, supercharged cells beginning in the early 20th century, but it was not until 1963 that stem cells were actually discovered. Canadian researchers at the Ontario Cancer Institute in Toronto were investigating the properties of bone marrow; specifically, they wanted to know how injections of marrow would affect laboratory mice that had undergone lethal doses of radiation. The lead researchers, Ernest McCulloch and James Till, found that the injections caused the mice to develop nodules on the spleen that were filled with white and red blood cells. After examining the cells under a microscope, McCulloch and Till observed that about 1 in 1,000 of the cells behaved differently from the others: not only could these unique cells reproduce indefinitely, they also had the ability to differentiate into a wide variety of new blood cells. Finally, the amazing properties of stem cells were understood, and McCulloch and Till became known as the fathers of stem cell research.

Ironically, stem cells had already been used in surgery years before McCulloch and Till made their discovery—but the doctor who performed the surgery did not know what he was dealing with. In the 1950s children who were diagnosed with leukemia (a cancer of the blood) were given an almost certain death sentence. Through experiments with animals, physician E. Donnall Thomas of New York had found that bone marrow contained something that helped regenerate blood and the immune system, although he had no way of knowing that "something"

> " Studies and experiments with adult stem cells have produced cures for diseases that were once thought to be untreatable, and certainly incurable. "

was stem cells. "We knew they were there," he says, "but we didn't know what they were. . . . Basically, we found we could inject bone marrow cells into patients without killing them. In retrospect, I'm surprised at how stupid we were."[16] In 1956, using bone marrow from an identical twin, Thomas performed a bone marrow transplant that saved the life of a leukemia patient. Even though he did not know the significance of the operation at the time, he had performed the world's first human stem cell transplant. Thirteen years later, Thomas again made medical history. After extensive work on tissue typing and development of antibiotics that would prevent transplant infections, he performed the first successful bone marrow transplant on a patient whose donor was not a twin.

Groundbreaking Research

Years after adult stem cells had been treating and curing people of disease, scientists were still struggling with embryonic stem cell research. In 1981 researchers from the United States and United Kingdom became the first to isolate and culture embryonic stem cells from mice, but accomplishing the same thing with human embryonic stem cells proved to be a daunting task. Researcher James A. Thomson performed many of his own experiments with mouse embryonic stem cells. He theorized, though, that the same mix of chemicals used to grow mouse stem cells in culture would not work with human embryonic stem cells. He explains: "If you compare a mouse embryo to a human embryo, they are as different as night and day. Even some of the molecules that control the embryo's development in the mouse are different or missing entirely in humans."[17] Thomson began working to perfect a cell culture recipe that could be used on a species closer to humans than the mouse. In 1995 he succeeded in creating the first embryonic stem cell line derived from monkeys.

> " Thomson concluded that [the embryonic stem cells] could be coaxed into becoming any type of tissue in the human body. "

Three years later, Thomson made an announcement that took the scientific world by storm—he had isolated human embryonic stem cells. Using spare embryos that had been donated for research by parents, he grew the microscopic orbs in culture dishes that contained his special nutrient solution. Within a few days they developed into blastocysts.

Peering through a microscope, Thomson used a very thin, hollow glass needle to extract the stem cells from their inner mass and then carefully placed the cells in a different chemical broth. The stem cells continued to divide and formed stem cell lines while still retaining their unspecialized state. When Thomson removed the cells from their culture dishes and injected them into mice, the cells divided rapidly and formed teratomas that contained bits of skin, muscle, and bone. Close examination of the cells showed that they were indeed embryonic stem cells, and Thomson concluded that they could be coaxed into becoming any type of tissue in the human body.

Scientific Breakthroughs

One of the most profound discoveries in stem cell research was announced in November 2007. Working independently in laboratories on two separate continents, scientists James A. Thomson of Wisconsin and Shinya Yamanaka of Kyoto University in Japan used ordinary human skin cells to grow stem cells. Using cells taken from the amputated foreskin of a newborn boy, Thomson's group added four genes to the cells, which reprogrammed them to become induced pluripotent stem (ISP) cells—and they were essentially identical to embryonic stem cells in function and biological structure. Yamanaka's group used the same procedure, reprogramming skin cells that were taken from the face of a 36-year-old woman.

Although this technique is in its earliest stages of development, scientists throughout the world have called it one of the most exciting advancements in medicine. In February 2008 a team of researchers at the University of California at Los Angeles announced that they, too, had reprogrammed skin cells to create ISP cells, and others will undoubtedly follow suit.

Do Adult Stem Cells Have Untapped Potential?

Scientists are constantly making new and exciting discoveries about adult stem cells, and they are learning that the potential of these cells might be greater than was originally thought.

In 2006 researchers in the United Kingdom took stem cells from the retinas of newborn mice and transplanted them into the eyes of mice that had lost their vision. The cells connected with existing cells and the creatures were able to see again. Andrew Dick, an ophthalmology professor at the University of Bristol, explains his reaction to the discovery: "As with any basic research we have to be careful not to overhype. However, this is a stunning piece of research that may in the distant future lead to transplants in humans to relieve blindness."[18]

Researchers have also learned that adult stem cells are contained in many more areas of body tissue than was originally believed—and some of these stem cells are capable of undergoing transformations into a variety of tissue types. Researchers at Northwestern University discovered that human megakaryocytes, or bone marrow cells that produce blood platelets, could be reprogrammed into cells that are similar to infection-fighting white blood cells.

> " Scientists are constantly making new and exciting discoveries about adult stem cells, and they are learning that the potential of these cells might be greater than was originally thought. "

Hair follicles have also been proven to contain adult stem cells. In 2006 researchers at the University of Pennsylvania School of Medicine used scalp tissue obtained from a national tissue network and isolated the stem cells. They grew the cells in culture and then differentiated them into nerve cells, smooth muscle cells, and skin pigment cells known as melanocytes. According to senior researcher George Xu, the team was excited to learn that the stem cells showed potential for a large variety of applications. "Although we are just at the start of this research," Xu says, "our findings suggest that human hair follicles may provide an accessible, individualized source of stem cells."[19] Stem cells from hair follicles are also being used by researchers in Leipzig, Germany. They have developed a method of growing the stem cells in culture and coaxing them to become skin cells, which they use to create skin grafts for patients with severe burns or other wounds. Currently these conditions are treated by grafting on the patient's own skin, usually taken from the thigh, but this creates scarring on the thigh as well as the treated area. Researchers say that the new technique will achieve the same result without scarring, and they believe they will be able to grow skin grafts for 10 to 20 patients a month.

Another breakthrough stem cell discovery was made by researchers at the University of California at Los Angeles, who transformed ordinary human fat cells into smooth muscle cells. The researchers, led by Dr. Larissa V. Rodriguez, first cultured the fat cells in a special chemical solution that encouraged them to grow into muscle cells. Then they tested the cells to see if they would expand and contract like smooth muscle tissue, and found that their efforts had been successful. To ensure that they would be able to reproduce the smooth muscle cells, they cloned one of the stem cells and again succeeded in producing muscle cells with a cloned cell population. The reason this discovery is so promising is because of the importance of smooth muscle cells to the human body. They help with normal function of numerous organs such as the intestines, bladder, and arteries; although they have also been produced from stem cells in the brain and bone marrow, acquiring them from fat is easier because most patients have fatty tissue readily available. According to Rodriguez, the study may help researchers learn how to use fat stem cells for smooth muscle tissue engineering and repair.

> **According to Atala . . . if 100,000 pregnant women donated their amniotic cells for research, this would provide enough genetically diverse cells for all the tissue needed by everyone in the country.**

Stem Cells from Pregnant Moms

Scientists who tout the superiority of embryonic stem cells cite their pluripotency, which makes them much more versatile than adult stem cells. But a discovery announced in January 2007 offered great promise for stem cells found in amniotic fluid, which surrounds and protects a developing fetus in the womb. The stem cells are easy to harvest from fluid left over from amniocentesis tests, which are often given to pregnant women. A research team led by Anthony Atala, director of the

Wake Forest University School of Medicine's Institute for Regenerative Medicine, announced that amniotic fluid stem cells share the versatility of embryonic cells, including pluripotency. These newly discovered stem cells appear to have the same potential as embryonic stem cells to become any of each of the more than 200 cell types in the human body. Atala explains: "So far, we've been successful with every cell type we've attempted to produce from these stem cells."[20] The team coaxed the stem cells to become brain cells as well as cells from the heart muscle, blood vessels, fat, nerves, and liver tissue. Under other conditions cells differentiated into osteoblasts, which build and strengthen bone. When the osteoblasts were implanted in mice, they formed a healthy tissue that was stronger and denser than normal mouse bone—and unlike embryonic stem cells, the amniotic cells did not cause tumors. Another exciting finding was that the amniotic stem cells grew just as fast as embryonic stem cells, doubling about every 36 hours. According to Atala, there are approximately 4 million births in the United States each year. If 100,000 pregnant women donated their amniotic cells for research, this would provide enough genetically diverse cells for all the tissue needed by everyone in the country.

"Our Acts and Efforts Generate Hope"

Scientists and others who are enthusiastic about stem cell research are looking toward the future. They realize that, as with any new type of medical science, success cannot happen overnight. Progress will be slow and there will be failures along the way, but they are convinced that the research must continue. Christopher Thomas Scott says that people who are against stem cell research often fear any type of biomedical science that seems to move too fast and intrudes into the natural world. They fear that "sooner or later, there will be no mysteries left to solve. On that day, we will lose our innocence, and perhaps our humanity." Yet Scott goes on to say that scientists must continue to pursue knowledge that holds promise for improving human health. "We do so because our acts and efforts generate hope—hope for legions of parents, children, husbands, wives, and friends who need those cures. The optimism that we can improve life and relieve suffering *is* our humanity."[21]

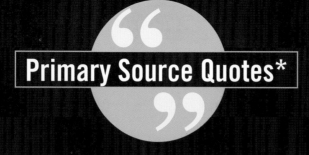

Primary Source Quotes*

Is Stem Cell Research Necessary?

66 **Stem cells of both varieties show enormous promise for seemingly miraculous medical treatments, from reversing the effects of Alzheimer's disease to repairing a damaged spinal cord.** 99

—Steven Edwards, "Thousands of Adult Stem Cell Deaths Show Urgency of Embryonic Research," *Wired*, April 11, 2007. www.wired.com.

Edwards, who writes for the *Wired Science* blog, is a strong advocate of stem cell research.

66 **Stem cells have been promoted as a cure for numerous diseases in the popular press, although the reality of the science suggests otherwise.** 99

—Rich Deem, "What Is Wrong with Embryonic Stem Cell Research?" God and Science, November 23, 2007. www.godandscience.org.

Deem works at Cedars-Sinai Medical Center's Davis Research Institute and runs the God and Science Web site.

Bracketed quotes indicate conflicting positions.

* Editor's Note: While the definition of a primary source can be narrowly or broadly defined, for the purposes of Compact Research, a primary source consists of: 1) results of original research presented by an organization or researcher; 2) eyewitness accounts of events, personal experience, or work experience; 3) first-person editorials offering pundits' opinions; 4) government officials presenting political plans and/or policies; 5) representatives of organizations presenting testimony or policy.

66 There is a history of public concern and even revulsion when new medical breakthroughs are announced. Think about heart transplants, artificial hearts, and test tube babies. But we come to embrace them eventually. There may be a similar course for stem cells. 99

—Jeffrey Kahn, quoted in CNN.com, "Jeff Kahn: Debate over Ethics of Stem Cell Research," August 10, 2001. http://archives.cnn.com.

Kahn is the director of the Center for Bioethics at the University of Minnesota and a professor in the university's School of Medicine.

66 To get [federal funding for embryonic stem cell research], stem-cell advocates have pulled out all the stops: distorting the facts, exaggerating the promise of the research, and confusing the public debate. 99

—Eric Cohen, "Inflated Promise, Distorted Facts," *National Review*, May 25, 2004. www.nationalreview.com.

Cohen is editor of *The New Atlantis*, resident scholar at the Ethics and Public Policy Center, and a consultant to the President's Council on Bioethics.

66 Stem cell research has the potential to affect the lives of millions of people in the United States and around the world. 99

—Bert Vogelstein, quoted in preface to *Stem Cells and the Future of Regenerative Medicine*, 2002.

Vogelstein is a noted cancer researcher with the Johns Hopkins University School of Medicine.

66 The assertion that embryonic stem cells . . . can be induced to form all the cells comprising the mature human body has been repeated so often that it seems incontrovertibly true. What is missing from this assertion remains the simple fact that there is essentially no scientific evidence supporting it. 99

—Maureen L. Condic, "What We Know About Embryonic Stem Cells," *First Things: The Journal of Religion, Culture, and Public Life*, January 2007. www.firstthings.com.

Condic is an associate professor of neurobiology and anatomy at the University of Utah School of Medicine.

❝ The first press reports on these [stem cell research facilities in New Jersey] won't be about amazing medical breakthroughs, but rather allegations of dubious research projects, dramatically overpaid researchers, and cozy contracts with the politically well-connected. ❞

—Gregg Edwards, "The Stem Cell Referendum: Politics Masquerading as Science," *NJ Voices*, NJ.com, November 2, 2007. http://blog.nj.com.

Edwards is president of the Center for Policy Research of New Jersey.

....

❝ For reasons that have more to do with politics than science, human embryonic stem-cell research attracts claims—pro and con—that stretch the imagination, if not the truth. ❞

—Tom Still, "Separating Hope from Hype in Stem-Cell Research," *Wisconsin Technology Network News*, July 6, 2007. http://wistechnology.com.

Still is president of the Wisconsin Technology Council and the former associate editor of the *Wisconsin State Journal* in Madison.

....

❝ Rockefeller University scientists are conducting basic research to improve scientific understanding of the biology of stem cells . . . [which] is crucial for the development of new treatments for diabetes, cancer, heart disease, stroke, spinal cord injury and such neurodegenerative disorders as Parkinson's and Alzheimer's diseases. ❞

Rockefeller University, "Stem Cell Research at the Rockefeller University," March 15, 2005. www.rockefeller.edu.

Located in New York City, the Rockefeller University is a world-renowned research institution.

....

❝I just don't see how we can turn our backs on this. . . . We have lost so much time already. I just really can't bear to lose any more.❞

—Nancy Reagan, quoted in BBC News, "Nancy Reagan Plea on Stem Cells," May 10, 2004. http://news.bbc.co.uk.

Reagan is the widow of Ronald Reagan, former president of the United States, who died of Alzheimer's disease in June 2004.

❝If the current controversy [over stem cell research] were to cause us to precipitously abandon this exciting area, it would be a catastrophic shame.❞

—David A. Shaywitz, "Stem Cell Hype and Hope," *Washington Post*, January 12, 2006. www.washingtonpost.com.

Shaywitz is an endocrinologist at the Harvard Stem Cell Institute.

❝So let's just give [embryonic stem cell] researchers all the money they want for their decades away promise, mindful that those funds could have gone to [adult stem cell] research projects treating and curing humans today. Then perhaps they'll announce that, given enough money and perhaps decades, they'll also build a computer with the processing power of a dime-store calculator.❞

—Michael Fumento, "Adult Approaches: Will Embryonic Stem Cell Promise Ever Pay Off?" *American Spectator*, May 2007. www.fumento.com.

Fumento is a Washington, D.C.–based health, science, and military writer and the author of numerous books.

Is Stem Cell Research Necessary?

- The human body is made up of **trillions of cells** of more than **200 types**; all these cells are produced by stem cells.

- Three- to five-day-old embryos (known as blastocysts) contain about **200 stem cells**.

- **Embryonic stem cells** are **pluripotent**, meaning they can form every type of cell in the body with the exception of placenta.

- **Adult stem cells are multipotent**, or capable of changing into limited types of cells.

- Adult stem cells are found throughout the body tissue of **children and adults**.

- In the laboratory, scientists are able to differentiate between stem cells and ordinary adult blood cells by using molecules that recognize and attach to specific surface proteins and that can **fluoresce** under certain **wavelengths of light**.

- By implanting human stem cells that lead to a particular disease into a mouse blastocyst, researchers can study when and how the **afflicted cells** begin to show signs of **disease** and **test drugs** that might prevent the onset of disease.

Stem Cells and Cloning

A stem cell is an unspecialized cell that can be encouraged to grow into a specialized type of cell. Many researchers believe that there is great hope for somatic cell nuclear transfer (SCNT), the scientific term for cloning. SCNT involves creating cloned embryos in order to harvest the stem cells that develop inside them. Scientists have successfully cloned embryos, but no one yet has been able to produce stem cells from them.The following illustrates how SCNT works, and how stem cells could theoretically be removed and grown into cloned stem cell lines.

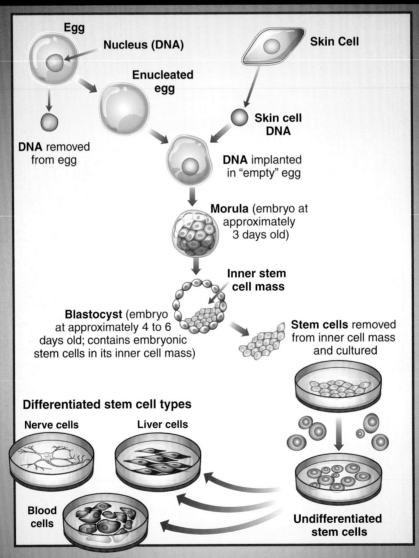

Source: "Understanding Stem Cells," The National Academies, October 2006. http://dels.nas.edu.

Where Adult Stem Cells Are Found in Humans

Researchers once thought that adult stem cells were only found in bone marrow and a few other select areas of the body. In recent years, however, they have learned that stem cells are found throughout the body and are far more plentiful than what was originally thought. The following illustration shows other areas where stem cells are found.

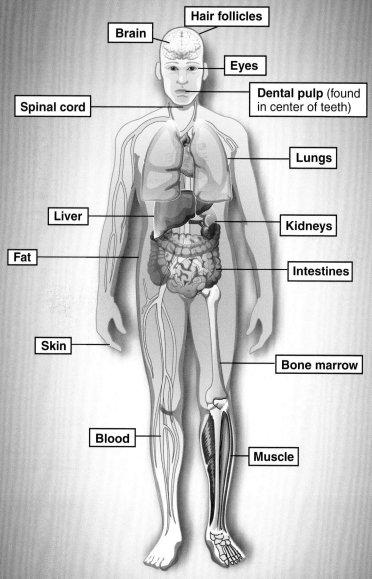

Hair follicles

Brain

Eyes

Spinal cord

Dental pulp (found in center of teeth)

Lungs

Liver

Kidneys

Fat

Intestines

Skin

Bone marrow

Blood

Muscle

Sources: Christopher Thomas Scott, *Stem Cell Now*, p. 66; "Understanding Stem Cells," The National Academies, October 2006; http://dels.nas.edu; Michael Fumento, "Adult Approaches: Will Embryonic Stem Cell Promise Ever Pay Off?" *American Spectator*, May 2007. www.fumento.com.

Stem Cells in Bone Marrow

Over the years, stem cell research has resulted in an astounding number of discoveries. Since the 1960s, scientists have known that a rich source of adult stem cells can be found in bone marrow, the soft, spongy tissue inside bone cavities. The stem cells in bone marrow produce red blood cells to carry oxygen throughout the body, white blood cells to fight off infection, and tiny blood-clotting cells known as platelets.

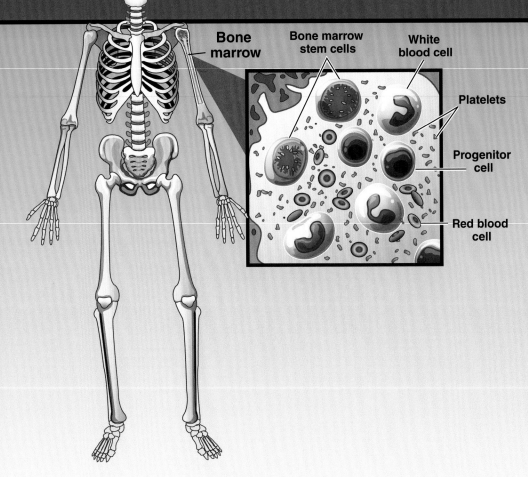

Bone marrow

Bone marrow stem cells

White blood cell

Platelets

Progenitor cell

Red blood cell

Sources: Janet Basu, "Genes, Stem Cells and Bone Marrow Transplants," *UCSF Magazine*, May 2003. http://publ.ucsf.edu/magazine; "Bone Marrow Transplant," National Institutes of Health, October 30, 2006. www.nlm.nih.gov; Christopher Thomas Scott, *Stem Cell Now*. New York: Penguin, 2006, p. 67.

Public Viewpoints About Stem Cell Research

In November/December 2007, Virginia Commonwealth University conducted a survey of 1,000 adults throughout the United States. Respondents were asked a series of questions about their views on stem cell research.

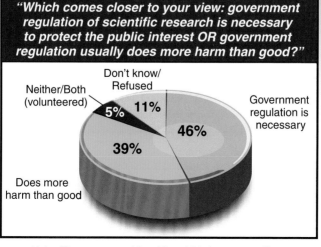

"Scientific research is essential for improving the quality of human lives."

Disagree **2%** Don't know/Refused
7%
30% **62%**
Agree somewhat
Agree strongly

"New technology used in medicine allows people to live longer and better."

Disagree **2%** Don't know/Refused
9%
33% **57%**
Agree strongly
Agree somewhat

"Which comes closer to your view: government regulation of scientific research is necessary to protect the public interest OR government regulation usually does more harm than good?"

Don't know/ Refused
Neither/Both (volunteered)
5% **11%** **46%**
39%
Government regulation is necessary
Does more harm than good

Note: Figures may add to 99 or 101 due to rounding.

Source: "VCU Life Sciences Survey 2007," Virginia Commonwealth University, December 2007. www.vcu.edu.

Is Stem Cell Research Ethical?

> **The possible benefits for treating a variety of illnesses outweigh the political and religious concerns that for too long have stymied research in the U.S.**
>
> —*Seattle Times*, editorial, "Stem-Cell Developments Are Not Replacements."

> **The production and destruction of human embryos required for embryonic stem cell research is a significant ethical and moral problem. Human beings, even the tiniest developing human beings, should not be used in experiments which result in their death.**
>
> —Richard A. Chole and Barbara Quigley, "The Facts on Cloning & Stem Cell Research."

O n July 19, 2006, when President George W. Bush gave a speech about stem cell research, he was surrounded by families with small children. He purposely asked that these families be present because the children had been born after being adopted as embryos. Bush was making the point that no matter how tiny and undeveloped embryos are, they are undeniably human and to destroy them on behalf of science is unethical and wrong. "Each of these children began his or her life as a frozen embryo that was created for in vitro fertilization, but remained unused after the fertility treatments were complete," said Bush.

> Each of these children was adopted while still an embryo, and has been blessed with the chance to grow up in a loving family. These boys and girls are not spare parts. They

remind us of what is lost when embryos are destroyed in the name of research. They remind us that we all begin our lives as a small collection of cells. And they remind us that in our zeal for new treatments and cures, America must never abandon our fundamental morals.[22]

The belief that destroying human embryos is akin to murder is the most common argument made by opponents of embryonic stem cell research—yet the debate does not stop there. The entire field of stem cell research is fraught with ethical considerations, from embryo destruction to genetic engineering and SCNT cloning. People have a wide range of perspectives about what is right and what is wrong, and while their viewpoints differ radically from each other, they all share one undeniable trait: passion for what they believe in.

Are Embryos Equal to People?

Of all the diverse opinions about stem cell research, the most contentious disagreements are over human embryos; specifically, whether anyone has the right to destroy them to harvest their stem cells. Opponents of this research argue that embryos are a form of life that can potentially develop into children—that every man, woman, and child on earth started out the exact same way. Why, they ask, should embryos be treated with less respect and dignity than developed human beings? Even many advocates of embryonic stem cell research are somewhat torn over the issue, as Christopher Thomas Scott writes: "Embryonic stem cells touch us deeply, not just because they might cure disease. It is because forms of human life are at stake—living embryos and living persons."[23]

No one could disagree that human embryos have the potential to become children. But most supporters of embryonic stem cell research believe that *potential* is not the same as *actual,* and that an embryo is not the equivalent of a human being until it has been implanted in a mother's womb. Harvard University researcher Doug Melton used donated embryos to produce new lines of stem cells in 2004. He takes issue with people who believe that life begins at conception, as he explains:

> Unquestionably, the material from which these stem cells are derived has the potential to form a life. But this potential is very low. Those who say that frozen embryos

are identical to children are mistaken. You cannot take a child and put it in a freezer. We need to draw a strong line between what has the potential for life and what is alive. Even more important, the material we used was slated for destruction. From that point of view, one could almost consider our position pro-life. We took something that was going to be destroyed and isolated cells from it that could improve the lives of people suffering from disease and trauma. I don't know of any scientist who thinks this was a bad idea or that it should not have been done.[24]

Proponents of embryonic stem cell research share Melton's opinion about putting embryos to good use rather than destroying them. One is Orrin Hatch, a Republican U.S. senator and staunch right-to-life advocate who has surprised and dismayed many of his fellow conservatives because of his views on embryonic stem cells. Hatch rejects the notion that embryonic stem cell research is unethical or immoral. "The reality today," he says, "is that each year thousands of embryos are routinely destroyed. Why shouldn't embryos slated for destruction be used for the benefit of mankind?"[25]

> **The belief that destroying human embryos is akin to murder is the most common argument made by opponents of embryonic stem cell research—yet the debate does not stop there.**

Another question raised by embryonic stem cell advocates is, if embryos should not be destroyed for their stem cells, then where is the outrage over the thousands of embryos that are destroyed every year by fertility clinics? And if embryos are the moral equivalent of human beings, why are politicians not lobbying to ban all means of destroying them, rather than just focusing on those that are used for research? According to Harvard political philosophy professor Michael J. Sandel, this is flawed reasoning that makes no sense. He explains:

If embryos are human beings, to allow fertility clinics to

discard them is to countenance, in effect, the widespread creation and destruction of surplus children. Those who believe that a blastocyst is morally equivalent to a baby must believe that the 400,000 excess embryos languishing in freezers in US fertility clinics are like newborns left to die by exposure on a mountainside. But those who view embryos in this way should not only be opposing embryonic stem cell research; they should also be leading a campaign to shut down what they must regard as rampant infanticide in fertility clinics.[26]

An Ethical Compromise?

Researchers have developed a new technique for creating stem cells that many people, including some who are opposed to embryonic stem cell research, believe is a more ethical approach. In January 2008 scientist Robert Lanza announced that he and a team of researchers had created viable new lines of embryonic stem cells from human embryos that were not destroyed. The technique, known as blastomere biopsy, involved taking a single cell from a two-day-old embryo and growing it in a special culture to coax it to become an embryonic stem cell. According to Lanza, more than 80 percent of the embryos from which the cells were removed grew into healthy blastocysts. Scientists are excited about the discovery because its potential is so promising. Fertility doctors commonly remove a single cell from a young embryo and test it for genetic defects before implanting it in a woman's womb. These

> " Another question raised by embryonic stem cell advocates is, if embryos should not be destroyed for their stem cells, then where is the outrage over the thousands of embryos that are destroyed every year by fertility clinics? "

"spare" cells could conceivably be used to grow new stem cell lines—and could significantly increase the number of stem cells needed for research without destroying embryos.

Lanza and other scientists are hopeful that the new technique will sidestep the ethical issues of embryonic stem cell research and become eligible for federal monies. Their hopes were given a boost when the National Institutes of Health (NIH) announced that blastomere biopsy was "a potential source of ethically acceptable embryonic stem cells."[27] Once the agency has thoroughly reviewed the technique, it will make a formal recommendation on whether the technique should receive federal research funding.

"We Don't Want to Create Frankenstein"

Making cloned embryos for research purposes is not the biggest source of controversy in the stem cell debate, but it is a contentious issue nevertheless. Some are convinced that in the same way it is wrong to destroy an embryo for its stem cells, intentionally creating a cloned embryo that is designed to be destroyed for its stem cells is equally wrong. Another factor is that many people do not understand the difference between SCNT cloning and reproductive cloning. The process for each is much the same: the nucleus of a female's egg is removed and replaced with the nucleus of a cell from a different female or male. Yet the end result is markedly different. SCNT involves the creation of human embryos strictly for use in research (research cloning) and eventually for therapeutic purposes (therapeutic cloning). In reproductive cloning, the embryo is implanted in a womb so it can grow into a living animal. In 1996 scientists from Edinburgh, Scotland, used this technique to create Dolly the sheep, the world's first cloned mammal. Since that time, other types of animals have been cloned, including cows, goats, pigs, rats, mice, rabbits, cats, dogs, and mules. Animal cloning is considered acceptable by many scientists, but human reproductive cloning is widely condemned, as Scott writes: "Attempting to . . . use embryos to make fetuses or human beings for spare parts would amount to the worst

> " Making cloned embryos for research purposes is not the biggest source of controversy in the stem cell debate, but it is a contentious issue nevertheless. "

forms of illegal and unethical human experimentation. Our moral codes are designed to protect people in our pursuit of knowledge, and humans or fetuses cloned for research purposes fall squarely and unambiguously into this category."[28]

Even though SCNT is not intended to make cloned human beings, some people argue that any type of cloning should be banned. In their view, cloning is a sign that science has clearly gone too far. That is the perspective of Charles Krauthammer, a psychiatrist and syndicated columnist who is a member of the President's Council on Bioethics. Krauthammer fears that some researchers may be tempted to use unscrupulous methods to create human clones that would be used for harvesting tissues, organs, and other vital body parts whenever they were needed. He explains: "We will, slowly and by increments, have gone from stem cells to embryo farms to factories with fetuses hanging (metaphorically) on meat hooks waiting to be cut open and used by the already born."[29]

Those who do not share this perspective typically become frustrated, saying that the research is vital and warranted and must be pursued. This is often the case with people who are suffering from chronic diseases or injuries, as well as their family members. Michael J. Fox, a well-known actor and advocate of all types of stem cell research, decries this sort of argument against cloning. He explains: "It's ridiculous. It's so self-defeating for those of us with Parkinson's and other degenerative diseases. We don't want to create Frankenstein or clone our Uncle Charlie so we can play poker with him again. It's nuts. We just want to save lives."[30]

"Savior Babies"

Molly Nash is a girl from Colorado who is alive because of stem cell research—but the circumstances leading up to her life-saving operation created a major ethical controversy. Molly was born in 1994 with a rare genetic blood disease known as Fanconi anemia. Her prognosis was grim, as most children stricken with it develop leukemia and die at a young age. The disease can be cured by a matching bone marrow transplant from a healthy sibling, but Molly was an only child. Her parents were both carriers of the gene that causes Fanconi anemia, and while they desperately wanted more children, they feared that a second baby would also be born with the deadly disease. The Nashes decided to conceive through in vitro fertilization, and then undergo preimplantation genetic diagnosis (or

PGD), a procedure used to detect abnormalities and genetic matches in embryos. A total of 24 embryos were created; genetic screening showed that one was free of Fanconi anemia as well as a perfect match for Molly. The embryo was implanted in the mother's womb, and 9 months later, a healthy, robust baby boy named Adam was born. When he was 5 weeks old, doctors at the University of Minnesota transplanted stem cells from his umbilical cord blood into his sister. Today, although some symptoms of her disease remain, Molly is a healthy teenage girl.

Although Molly's story had a happy ending, many people are disturbed by the very idea of PGD because of its ethical implications. The embryos are created for specific reasons, and those that are not needed are discarded as medical waste. This, opponents say, greatly devalues human life and allows parents to pick and choose from embryos for whatever reason, from gender selection to physical characteristics. Ethicist John F. Kilner of the Center for Bioethics and Human Dignity shares his thoughts: "Helping sick children is wonderful and should be a high priority. We ache with their parents and are motivated to do all that we can to help. But once we suggest that accomplishing something good can be pursued using any means necessary, we have crossed an ethical line." Kilner calls the children intentionally created for a specific purpose "Savior Babies" and adds that "allowing human beings to live only if they 'measure up' genetically represents a profound shift in what it means to be a human being. It suggests that some human beings do not have enough value to justify their existence."[31]

The War Between Ethics and Science

The controversy over stem cell research continues to rage on, and it is not a simple problem to overcome. Even researchers who support embryonic stem cell research and SCNT cloning are often troubled by the ethical issues. Thomson, who is a supporter of all types of stem cell research, still finds embryo destruction to be a moral dilemma—one that he has struggled with since he first isolated human embryos in 1998. He shares his thoughts: "If human embryonic stem cell research does not make you at least a little bit uncomfortable, you have not thought about it enough. I thought long and hard about whether I would do it."[32]

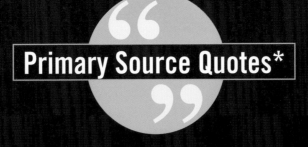

❝I come to this issue as a proud right-to-life senator. I do believe, very strongly, that it is possible to be both anti-abortion and pro-embryonic stem cell research. I believe that pro-life means caring for the living as well.❞

—Orrin Hatch, quoted in Raymond J. Keating, "The Politics of Embryonic Stem Cell Research," *Orthodoxy Today*, May 21, 2005. www.orthodoxytoday.org.

Hatch is a U.S. senator representing Utah.

❝Destroying human life in the hopes of saving human life is not ethical—and it is not the only option before us.❞

George W. Bush, quoted in Doug Trapp, "Bush Rejects Second Stem Cell Bill; Veto Override Is Unlikely," *AMNews*, July 9, 2007. www.ama-assn.org.

Bush is the forty-third president of the United States.

Bracketed quotes indicate conflicting positions.

* Editor's Note: While the definition of a primary source can be narrowly or broadly defined, for the purposes of Compact Research, a primary source consists of: 1) results of original research presented by an organization or researcher; 2) eyewitness accounts of events, personal experience, or work experience; 3) first-person editorials offering pundits' opinions; 4) government officials presenting political plans and/or policies; 5) representatives of organizations presenting testimony or policy.

❝ Imagine that you have a house that is on fire. You have two children, the family dog and some embryos frozen in the cellar. Whom would you rescue first? Most people would rescue their children first. Then whom would you rescue? Would you rescue the frozen embryos or the family dog? I'm not trying to make light of this, but most people would probably rescue the dog. **❞**

—R. Michael Roberts, quoted in Mark Esser, "Stem Cell: No Simple Division," *Columbia Missourian*, October 29, 2006. www.columbiamissourian.com.

Roberts is professor of animal sciences at the University of Missouri.

❝ Implanting cloned embryos into a woman would occur in the privacy of the doctor-patient relationship, and once a mother has a clonal pregnancy, what will law enforcement do? . . . The only way to prevent baby cloning is to stop the process at the creation of cloned embryos. **❞**

—David Christensen, "Patients, Not Politics," *National Review*, June 7, 2007.

Christensen is director of congressional affairs at the Family Research Council.

❝ There's a world of difference between reproductive cloning—something that should be banned right away—and therapeutic cloning. Therapeutic cloning offers great promise for curing deadly and terrible diseases. SCNT saves lives; it doesn't create lives. **❞**

—Christopher and Dana Reeve Foundation, "Somatic Cell Nuclear Transfer: SCNT 101," 2007. www.christopherreeve.org.

The Christopher and Dana Reeve Foundation, started by the late Christopher Reeve, is dedicated to curing spinal cord injury and improving the quality of life for people living with paralysis.

66 We oppose embryonic stem cell research because it destroys the embryo. . . . It doesn't make any difference if it's in a petri dish, implanted in the womb or in a nursery. A human life is a human life. Are we going to say a 4-year-old is more human than a 2-year-old? 99

—Pam Fichter, quoted in Peter Slevin, "In the Heartland, Stem Cell Research Meets Fierce Opposition," *Washington Post*, August 10, 2005. www.washingtonpost.com.

Fichter is president of Missouri Right to Life.

66 Embryonic stem-cell research is another issue where conservatives have latched onto fringe science in order to advance moral arguments. 99

—Chris Mooney, "Research and Destroy," *Washington Monthly*, October 2004.

Mooney is senior correspondent for the *American Prospect* magazine and the author of two books.

66 Saying that a human embryo is not a person because it is not fully developed is very dangerous reasoning. I'm 68 years old and I'm not fully developed, I will still learn new things and new skills. I'm afraid that if we apply this reasoning to other situations, we could say that a lot of people could be sacrificed for not being fully developed. 99

—James Sowash, quoted in Mark Esser, "Stem Cell: No Simple Division," *Columbia Missourian*, October 29, 2006. www.columbiamissourian.com.

Sowash is a retired physician from Missouri.

66 Science is a gift of God to all of us and science has taken us to a place that is biblical in its power to cure. And that is the embryonic stem cell research. 99

—Nancy Pelosi, quoted in Jeff Zeleny, "House Votes to Expand Stem Cell Research," *New York Times*, June 8, 2007. www.nytimes.com.

Pelosi, a Democrat, is Speaker of the U.S. House of Representatives.

> **" Being pro-life is about more than caring for the un-born. It's about caring for the living as well. "**

—Christopher Murphy, quoted in Jeff Zeleny, "House Votes to Expand Stem Cell Research," *New York Times*, June 8, 2007. www.nytimes.com.

Murphy represents a district in the state of Connecticut in the U.S. House of Representatives.

> **" We don't think a human life should ever be a means to an end. It's not an ethical way to go about curing disease. "**

—Dennis Powst, quoted in Gail Robinson, "Stem Cell Research: Medical Miracle or Moral Morass?" *Gotham Gazette*, March 20, 2006. www.gothamgazette.com.

Powst is director of communications for the New York State Catholic Conference.

Facts and Illustrations

Is Stem Cell Research Ethical?

- **The first cloned mammal** was Dolly the sheep, created in 1996 by scientists in Scotland.

- Since the Snowflakes program was started by Nightlight Christian Adoptions in 1997, more than **130 embryos** have been adopted and are today healthy children.

- A December 2007 poll conducted by Virginia Commonwealth University showed that more than **50 percent** of the respondents believe scientific decisions should be based primarily on an analysis of the risks and benefits involved, while **32 percent** stated that morals and ethics should be primary considerations.

- A May 2006 poll by Opinion Research Corporation showed that **72 percent** of respondents favor embryonic stem cell research, which is up from **68 percent** in 2005.

- It can cost couples **$2,000** or more per year to keep their excess embryos frozen in fertility clinics, which is why many opt to have them destroyed; still, however, those who are opposed to embryonic stem cell research do not believe the embryos should be used for research.

- In 2005 the **National Academies** published **guidelines for scientists** who do research with human embryonic stem cells to encourage responsible and ethically sensitive conduct in their work.

Public Support for Embryonic Stem Cell Research Can Vary

When people participate in opinion polls, their responses often reflect how the questions are worded. For example, in a poll by the *Washington Post*, participants were asked: **"Do you support or oppose embryonic stem cell research?"** As the pie chart shows, 61 percent said they supported the research.

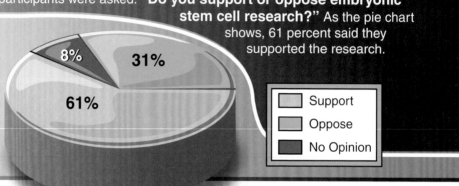

8%
31%
61%

Support
Oppose
No Opinion

The results of a poll by International Communications Research were quite different. The question asked these participants was, **"Stem cells are the basic cells from which all of a person's tissues and organs develop. Congress is considering the question of federal funding for experiments using stem cells from human embryos. The live embryos would be destroyed in their first week of development to obtain these cells. Do you support or oppose the use of federal tax dollars being used for such experiments?"** In this survey, only 38.6 percent said they supported the research.

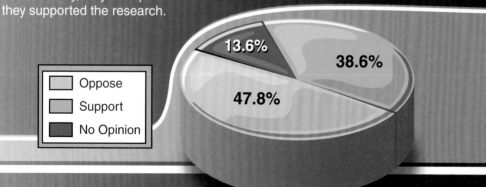

13.6%
38.6%
47.8%

Oppose
Support
No Opinion

Sources: Ruy Teixeira, "Public Opinion Snapshot: Solid Backing for Embryonic Stem Cell Research," Center for American Progress, March 30, 2007. www.americanprogress.org; "New Poll: Americans Continue to Oppose Funding Stem Cell Research That Destroys Human Embryos," United States Conference of Catholic Bishops, May 31, 2006. www.usccb.org.

State Policies on Embryonic Stem Cell Research

Some states have laws in place that restrict the use of human embryos in stem cell research, and six states (Arkansas, Indiana, Louisiana, Michigan, North Dakota, and South Dakota) ban it altogether. The map below shows how various states regulate stem cell research.

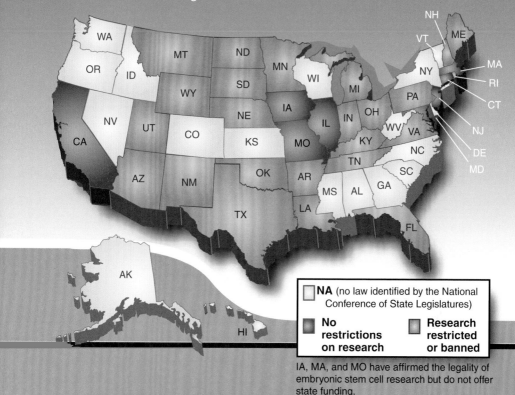

Legend:

☐ **NA** (no law identified by the National Conference of State Legislatures)

■ **No restrictions on research**

▨ **Research restricted or banned**

IA, MA, and MO have affirmed the legality of embryonic stem cell research but do not offer state funding.

Source: National Conference of State Legislatures, "Stem Cell Research," January 2008. www.ncsl.org.

- When **human and animal cells are mixed** in the lab, chimeras are produced; some people believe that the creation of chimeras involving human cells for research is morally acceptable as long as the creature has no level of human consciousness.

- Research has shown that cells isolated from a mouse morula (developmental stage prior to the blastocyst) can give rise to embryonic stem cells while the remaining morula cells develop into a healthy mouse; since the **morula could potentially be harmed**, however, using this technique on human morulas is morally objectionable to some.

Moral and Ethical Considerations of Stem Cell Research

Of all the issues known to science, there is perhaps none more controversial than stem cell research. The two most widely debated aspects are research involving human embryonic stem cells and SCNT cloning. Below are select results from a Virginia Commonwealth University study conducted in 2007.

"Do you favor or oppose medical research that uses stem cells from sources that do NOT involve human embryos?"

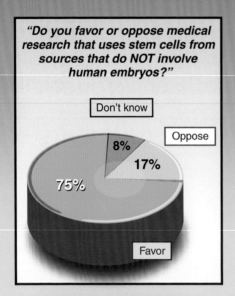

Don't know 8%
Oppose 17%
Favor 75%

"Do you favor or oppose using human cloning technology IF it is used ONLY to help medical research develop new treatments for disease?"

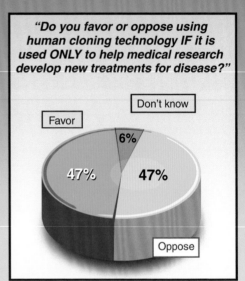

Favor 47%
Don't know 6%
Oppose 47%

"Should decisions about science and technology be based PRIMARILY on an analysis of the risks and benefits involved OR on the moral and ethical issues involved?"

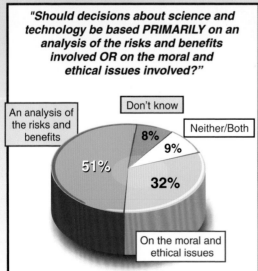

An analysis of the risks and benefits 51%
Don't know 8%
Neither/Both 9%
On the moral and ethical issues 32%

"Scientific research these days doesn't pay enough attention to the moral values of society."

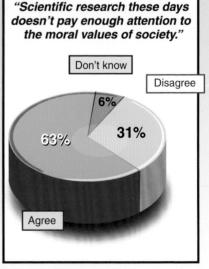

Don't know 6%
Disagree 31%
Agree 63%

Source: "VCU Life Sciences Survey 2007," Virginia Commonwealth University, December 2007. www.vcu.edu.

Donors Show Support For Embryonic Stem Cell Research

It is estimated that there are at least 400,000 embryos frozen at more than 400 fertility clinics throughout the United States. The media often refer to these embryos as "available for research," but that is not entirely true. Some donors are unwilling to donate their embryos for research. But a recent survey from Duke and Johns Hopkins Universities shows that a large percentage of donors with embryos currently frozen would be willing to allow them to be used in research.

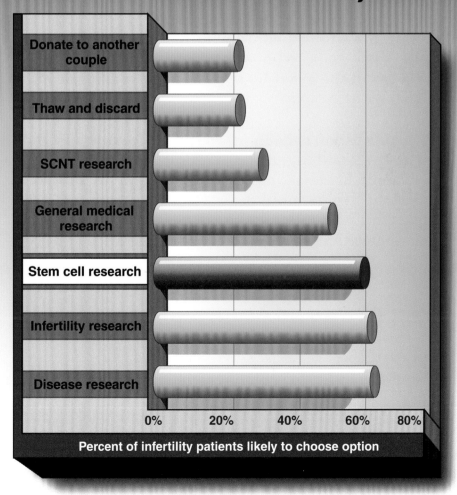

Intentions for Stored Embryos

Percent of infertility patients likely to choose option

Source: Anee Drapkin Lyerly and Ruth R. Faden, "Embryonic Stem Cells: Willingness to Donate Frozen Embryos for Stem Cell Research," *Science*, July 6, 2007. www.sciencemag.org.

Are Stem Cells the Answer to Prolonged Human Life?

❝Living, breathing people who have been treated by stem cells—some who would have otherwise died—are signs of the great hope of stem-cell research.❞

—David Christensen, "Patients, Not Politics."

❝The role of stem cells in medicine is already very real, but there is a danger of exaggerating the promise of new medical developments. What tend to be 'over-promised' are not only the potential outcomes of both embryonic and adult stem cell research, but also the time scales that are involved.❞

—National Academies, "Understanding Stem Cells."

Even with all that has been learned about stem cells throughout the years, the microscopic organisms are still mysterious to scientists. No one knows for sure why stem cells behave the way they do, what makes them differentiate, or why they divide and develop so vigorously when they are young and then stop growing when they get older. Another challenge for researchers is that stem cells are relatively unpredictable; they do not always act the way they are expected to during experiments. Although researchers gain more knowledge and understanding every day, much is still unknown. Still, most scientists are convinced that stem cells have immense potential to vastly improve human health and enable people to live longer, healthier lives.

The State of Human Health

Life expectancies have steadily risen since the early twentieth century. Whereas in 1930 the average life expectancy was only 59, today it is nearly 80. This is due in part to healthier lifestyles, improved sanitation, and better awareness of health-related issues, but much of the credit is due to revolutionary medical treatments and drugs. Years ago, if people of any age developed heart problems, cancer, serious blood disorders, or diseases of the liver or kidneys, they were most likely doomed to die. Now they have a better chance of being cured than ever before.

Yet deadly diseases still claim the lives of millions of people every year. In 2005 nearly 800,000 people in the United States died from heart disease and stroke. Heart disease is the leading cause of death in the United States, while diseases of the kidney and liver are among the top 15. Organ transplants can and do cure people of these diseases, but the need for healthy organs far surpasses the supply. According to the National Kidney Foundation, over 95,000 patients, 10 percent of whom are under the age of 18, need organ transplants—but in 2006 fewer than 29,000 transplants were performed, and more than 6,000 people died while waiting. With such grim statistics, it is no wonder that patients, families, doctors, and researchers look to stem cells as a way of vastly improving human health and saving people from disease.

The Power of Regeneration

In the animal kingdom, certain creatures have an amazing capability: newts, frogs, salamanders, worms, starfish, and tiny freshwater animals known as hydras are able to regrow organs and other parts of their bodies (in some cases, even heads) that have been injured or lost. This is possible because the creatures' stem cells have regenerative ability that far surpasses that of humans. Scientists from the University of Heidelberg in Germany explain: "Animals with staggering regenerative potential either have an abundance of stem cells or can de-differentiate specialized tissue cells into stem cells. . . . When they are in urgent need of a new limb, they convert adult differentiated cells back to an embryonic undifferentiated state. These cells then migrate to the site of injury where they regenerate the missing part."[33] Of course, humans cannot grow back amputated legs or arms or toes, but the stem cells in their bodies have powerful regenerative abilities. When someone is wounded or donates a pint of blood, the body replenishes the lost or damaged blood cells by drawing on hematopoietic cells that are contained in blood and bone marrow. After the surgical removal of half of someone's damaged liver, adult stem cells immediately start rebuilding the organ, and this repair may take only a few weeks. Other organs such as the lung, heart, and kidneys also have some capacity to repair themselves through regeneration.

Sometimes when organs are diseased or injured, their stem cells lose the ability to make the necessary repairs. That is why researchers are so enthusiastic about stem cell transplants and therapies; they believe that tissue damage could be reversed if lost or damaged cells were replaced with new cells. Science and health writer Eve Herold explains: "The principle behind stem cell research is that the formula for self-renewal, and for continuous cellular replenishment, hides within stem cells. . . . If we could unleash that regenerative power, control and direct it, we could cure or reverse a great many catastrophic diseases, injuries, and birth defects that are currently beyond the reach of medicine."[34]

> **Even with all that has been learned about stem cells throughout the years, the microscopic organisms are still mysterious to scientists.**

The regenerative ability of stem cells has already been proven with transplants and treatments using hematopoietic stem cells from bone marrow and umbilical cords, which currently treat about 80 different diseases. Studies with animals continue to show that stem cells have excellent potential for treating a wide variety of diseases and injuries. Scientists at Harvard Medical School implanted stem cells into the brains of mice with the kind of brain damage caused by strokes or cerebral palsy. The cells repaired the brains by replacing many of the missing nerve cells as well as protecting other cells from aging and dying. According to

Evan Snyder, a neurologist who led the research, this sort of repair could likely also take place in other organs such as the heart, lungs, and liver.

The regenerative power of stem cells transformed the life of a 65-year-old man from Finland. Because of the growth of a large benign tumor, his upper jaw had been removed, rendering him unable to eat or speak without a prosthesis. To make him a jaw, a team of researchers cultivated stem cells from his own fatty tissue and grew them for two weeks in a specially formulated solution that included his own blood serum. To shape the jaw, they built a scaffold out of biodegradable material and seeded it with the new cells. Then

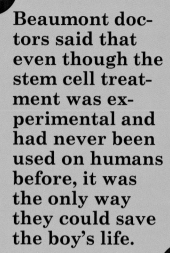

> **Beaumont doctors said that even though the stem cell treatment was experimental and had never been used on humans before, it was the only way they could save the boy's life.**

they implanted the scaffold in his abdomen so the cells and tissue could grow. Nine months later they removed the tissue-covered scaffold and transplanted it into his head. When the results of the procedure were announced in February 2008, researchers said that the man's face looked much the same as it had before his jaw had been removed.

A Lifesaving Treatment That Defied the Law

In the United States, bone marrow stem cells can be used to treat leukemia, immune deficiency disorders, and several other medical conditions, but the Food and Drug Administration prohibits them from being used to treat heart disease. In 2003, however, doctors at Beaumont Hospital in Royal Oak, Michigan, performed an emergency procedure that was not sanctioned by the FDA. In a freak accident, a 16-year-old boy named Dmitri Bonnville had been shot in the heart by an automatic nail gun, and a three-inch nail pierced one of his heart's main pumping chambers. Doctors removed the nail and patched the hole, but the boy suffered a massive heart attack that caused serious tissue damage. Fearing that the damage would soon spread to other areas of his heart, the doctors gave Dmitri a drug that would stimulate the production of bone marrow stem cells and their release into the bloodstream. Then they collected the stem cells and injected them into his heart. Follow-up tests showed that there was improvement in Dmitri's heart function, and six months after the treatment he was back in school and playing basketball with his friends. Beaumont doctors said that even though the stem cell treatment was experimental and had never been used on humans before, it was the only way they could save the boy's life.

Building Organs from Stem Cells

Because organs are in such short supply, one of scientists' greatest hopes is that stem cells will someday enable them to grow human organs. Although many people may consider such a feat as science fiction, animal and human organs are grown in laboratories all over the world, and scientists continue to make exciting progress in this area. In January 2008 researchers at the University of Minnesota announced that they had created a beating rat heart, which could pave the way toward the creation of human hearts and other vital organs. The team removed all the cells from the heart of a dead rat, leaving the valves and outer structure to serve as a scaffold for the new heart. They removed heart stem cells from newborn rats, placed the cells in the scaffold, and then stimulated them electronically to create artificial circulation to replicate blood pressure. Less than two weeks later the cells had mobilized to form the new beating heart, which was pumping a small amount of blood. When the heart was transplanted into a live rat, it began to grow and function normally. The lead researcher, Doris A. Taylor, says that her team "just took nature's own building blocks to build a new organ." She adds that the team was delighted with the results of their research: "The heart is a beautiful organ, and it's not one that I thought I'd ever be able to build in a dish." [35]

> " Because organs are in such short supply, one of scientists' greatest hopes is that stem cells will someday enable them to grow human organs. "

Researchers have also grown organs using human adult stem cells. In 2006 a research team from Great Britain used stem cells from umbilical cord blood to grow a human liver. They gathered the cells from cord blood and placed them in a device known as a bioreactor, which simulated weightlessness and helped the cells to multiply quickly. Then they added hormones and chemicals to turn the undifferentiated cells into liver cells. The researchers created several tiny livers, and they are optimistic that within several years they will be able to create large enough livers to be used in clinical trials.

Anthony Atala says that stem cells can also be used to "patch" diseased organs, promoting them to repair themselves. He scoffs at conventional medical beliefs that the only option is to replace organs, as he explains: "Why is it that surgeons think that if a piece of your heart gives out, you have to change the whole heart? You don't! Our organs have tremendous reserves. . . . You don't need much repair to get back to a normal lifestyle. And a stem cell patch may be the best approach."[36]

> " Today, researchers have a good understanding of what takes place in the brains of people who suffer from Parkinson's and Alzheimer's, but they still do not know what causes the diseases. "

Diseases That Destroy the Brain

When scientists talk about the vast potential of stem cells for treating humans, they often make reference to Parkinson's disease and Alzheimer's disease. These diseases, which claimed the lives of nearly 100,000 people in the United States during 2005, are progressive and incurable. Parkinson's disease occurs due to the gradual loss of nerve cells in particular areas of the brain. When these cells deteriorate and die, they stop producing a vital chemical known as dopamine, which is essential for proper functioning of the nervous system and smooth, coordinated muscle movement. As the disease progresses, patients develop uncontrollable tremors and spasms, rigidity of limbs, and abnormally decreased mobility.

Alzheimer's disease, which afflicts an estimated 50 percent of all people over the age of 85, is characterized by an abnormal buildup of proteins in the brain known as plaques and tangles. Early symptoms of

Alzheimer's include memory loss, confusion, poor judgment, and mood and personality changes. As the disease continues to progress it takes a devastating toll on the brain. Patients may hallucinate; develop increased memory loss; and have problems thinking, talking, and moving. The National Institute on Aging describes the final, most severe, phase: "In the last stage of AD, plaques and tangles are widespread throughout the brain, and areas of the brain have atrophied further. Patients cannot recognize family and loved ones or communicate in any way. They are completely dependent on others for care. All sense of self seems to vanish."[37]

Today, researchers have a good understanding of what takes place in the brains of people who suffer from Parkinson's and Alzheimer's, but they still do not know what causes the diseases. They hope that continued research with stem cells will increase their knowledge about these diseases and eventually lead to a cure. In studies with mice during 2002, MIT researchers found that implanted neural stem cells healed the injured nerve cells of aged mice whose brains were damaged by the equivalent of Parkinson's disease in humans. The researchers later said that early implantation of stem cells in humans could possibly forestall or even prevent degenerative brain diseases from forming.

Many scientists believe cloned embryonic stem cells have the potential to advance their understanding of Parkinson's and Alzheimer's. It is difficult for them to study the progression of these diseases in the brains of people suffering from them. But if some of the patients' damaged brain cells could be removed and used to clone stem cell lines, researchers could potentially trace the development of the diseases by watching how the cells behave in culture. Another possibility is that the cloned stem cell lines could be used to test drugs designed to regenerate lost nerves, rather than putting patients at risk by testing the drugs on humans.

Hope for the Future

The field of stem cell research still has many unknowns, and it will undoubtedly be years before diverse treatments and therapies are widely available for patients. But as research continues to reveal new and exciting developments, the idea that diseases and injuries can be treated and cured with stem cells becomes that much closer to reality.

Are Stem Cells the Answer to Prolonged Human Life?

66 Human embryonic stem (ES) cells capture the imagination because they are immortal and have an almost unlimited developmental potential. After many months of growth in culture dishes, these remarkable cells maintain the ability to form cells ranging from muscle to nerve to blood—potentially any cell type that makes up the body. 99

—Junying Yu and James A. Thomson, "Embryonic Stem Cells," *Regenerative Medicine*, National Institutes of Health, U.S. Department of Health and Human Services, August 2006. http://stemcells.nih.gov.

Yu and Thomson are researchers at the University of Wisconsin.

66 Isn't it time Americans recognize the promise of obtaining medical miracles from embryonic stem cells for the fairy tale it really is? 99

—Maureen L. Condic, "What We Know About Embryonic Stem Cells," *First Things: The Journal of Religion, Culture, and Public Life*, January 2007. www.firstthings.com.

Condic is an associate professor of neurobiology and anatomy at the University of Utah School of Medicine.

Bracketed quotes indicate conflicting positions.

* Editor's Note: While the definition of a primary source can be narrowly or broadly defined, for the purposes of Compact Research, a primary source consists of: 1) results of original research presented by an organization or researcher; 2) eyewitness accounts of events, personal experience, or work experience; 3) first-person editorials offering pundits' opinions; 4) government officials presenting political plans and/or policies; 5) representatives of organizations presenting testimony or policy.

66 **Stem cell research has the potential to cure more diseases than any other medical advance in recent memory—and perhaps in history altogether.** 99

—Sigrid Fry-Revere, "Best Hope Lies in Privately Funded Stem Cell Research," *Chicago Sun Times*, April 21, 2007.

Fry-Revere is the Cato Institute's director of bioethics studies.

66 **Provocative and conflicting claims have left the public (and most scientists) confused as to whether stem cell treatments are even medically feasible.** 99

—Robert Lanza and Nadia Rosenthal, "The Stem Cell Challenge: What Hurdles Stand Between the Promise of Human Stem Cell Therapies and Real Treatments in the Clinic?" *Scientific American*, May 24, 2004.

Lanza and Rosenthal are leading stem cell researchers.

66 **If scientists can figure out how to make viable embryonic stem cells from a clone, the human race would be a lot closer to personalized stem cell treatments, with new limbs and disease cures promised to anyone with a few spare skin flakes and enough money to foot the bill.** 99

—Brandon Keim, "Stem Cell Breakthrough, Sort of," *Wired Science*, January 17, 2008. http://blog.wired.com.

Keim is a freelance science and culture writer who lives in Brooklyn, New York.

66 If there is one message I can send to the research community it is this . . . prove to us that [stem cell technology] works. . . . Avoid hype and spin, tell us the truth, give us realistic expectations, and protect human subjects not because you have to, but because you want to. Then we in the patient community will be your strongest advocates. 99

—Abbey S. Meyers, "Unfulfilled Promises and Stem Cell Research," National Organization for Rare Disorders, November 20, 2001. www.rarediseases.org.

Meyers is president of the National Organization for Rare Disorders (NORD).

66 Recent developments in stem cell research may hold the key to improved treatments, if not cures, for those affected by Alzheimer's disease, diabetes, spinal cord injury and countless other conditions. 99

—Barack Obama, "Obama Renews Support for Embryonic Stem Cell Research," news release, April 11, 2007. http://obama.senate.gov.

Obama is a U.S. senator representing the state of Illinois.

66 From the scientific perspective, never believe anything until it's replicated several times. That's not an accusation of fraud, but science is full of honestly non-replicable findings. 99

—Hank Greely, quoted in Andy Coghlan, "'Hype' Accusation Blights Stem Cell Breakthrough," *New Scientist*, August 29, 2006. www.newscientist.com.

Greely is a professor at the Stanford University Law School who specializes in the legal implications of new biomedical technologies, including stem cells.

66 Those families who wake up every morning to face another day with a deadly disease or disability will not forget this decision by [President Bush] to stand in the way of sound science and medical research. 99

—Richard J. Durbin, quoted in Charles Babington, "Stem Cell Bill Gets Bush's First Veto," *Washington Post*, July 20, 2006. www.washingtonpost.com.

Durbin is a U.S. senator representing Illinois.

❝Leading scientists have told us time and time again that stem cell research . . . holds great promise in uncovering the mysteries of human health and disease and in potentially developing diagnostic tests and therapeutic agents for a multitude of conditions including cancer, heart disease, diabetes, Alzheimer's, Parkinson's and many, many others.❞

—Orrin Hatch, quoted in Adam Elggren, "Hatch: H.R. 810 Promotes Vital, Ethical Research," news release, July 13, 2005. http://hatch.senate.gov.

Hatch, a U.S. senator representing Utah, is a strong supporter of stem cell research.

❝Some prominent specialists . . . have said [embryonic stem cell therapy] is as many as 15 to 20 years away— and told me that the cells themselves may not become a treatment at all, but instead will point the way to other more efficient, cheaper approaches.❞

—Sally Lehrman, "Hope, Unfulfilled Promises on Stem Cell Work," *Boston Globe*, October 1, 2006. www.boston.com.

Lehrman reports on health and science issues for *Scientific American*, the radio program *The DNA Files*, and other media.

❝Stem cells can potentially be of enormous benefit for clinical treatment but as with the development of all drugs and therapies, there are safety issues that need to be investigated and resolved.❞

—Christopher Higgins, quoted in BBC News, "Adult Stem Cells 'Cancer Threat,'" April 20, 2005. http://news.bbc.co.uk.

Higgins is director of the Medical Research Council Clinical Science Centre in the United Kingdom.

Facts and Illustrations

Are Stem Cells the Answer to Prolonged Human Life?

- In 2005 nearly **800,000** people in the United States died of heart disease and stroke, over **500,000** died from cancer, nearly **75,000** died from diabetes, and nearly **100,000** died from Alzheimer's and Parkinson's disease.

- Heart disease is the **leading cause of death** in the United States.

- Currently, about **80 different diseases** are treated with adult stem cells from bone marrow and umbilical cord blood.

- The life expectancies of people diagnosed with leukemia, immune deficiency disorders, and other blood diseases have vastly increased because of treatments with **adult stem cells**.

- **Embryonic stem cells** have never been used in human experiments or treatments.

- Scientists have successfully **grown working organs** from animal and human stem cells.

- An estimated **95,000** people in the United States need organ transplants; in 2006 fewer than **29,000 transplants** were performed, and over **6,000 patients** died waiting.

The Promise of Stem Cell Research

Scientists are optimistic that stem cells will eventually lead to improved human health and prolonged life by aiding in drug development or correcting disease at the genetic level.

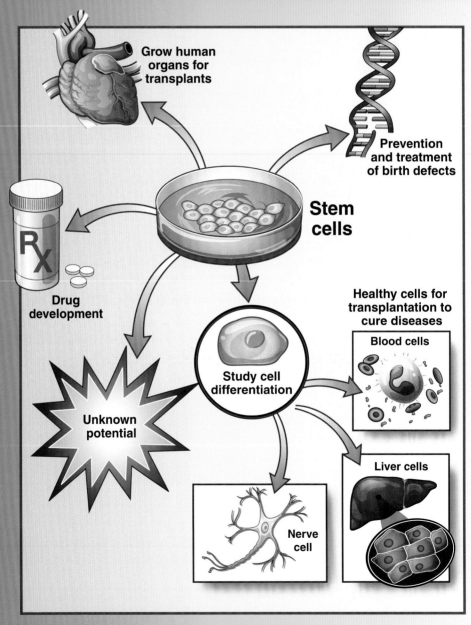

Grow human organs for transplants

Prevention and treatment of birth defects

Stem cells

Drug development

Healthy cells for transplantation to cure diseases

Blood cells

Study cell differentiation

Unknown potential

Liver cells

Nerve cell

Source: "Understanding Stem Cells," The National Academies, October 2006. http://dels.nas.edu.

Devastating Brain Diseases

Parkinson's and Alzheimer's are two degenerative brain diseases that killed nearly 100,000 people in the United States in 2005. Although scientists do not know what causes either disease, they have a good understanding of what takes place in the brains of people who suffer from them—and believe that stem cell research may hold the key to curing, and hopefully preventing, these devastating diseases. The following illustrations show the brain deterioration that is visible through Positron Emission Tomography (PET) scans in both diseases.

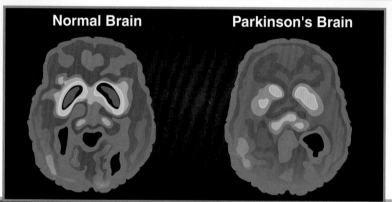

Normal Brain   **Parkinson's Brain**

Parkinson's occurs due to the gradual loss of nerve cells in particular areas of the brain. This halts the production of dopamine, a brain chemical that is essential for proper functioning of the nervous system and smooth, coordinated muscle movement. The above illustrations show the difference between a normal brain (left) and the brain of a Parkinson's patient (right).

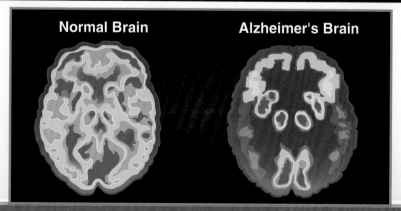

Normal Brain   **Alzheimer's Brain**

Alzheimer's is a fatal disease that is characterized by an abnormal buildup of proteins in the brain called plaques and tangles, which cause the brain to waste away over time. The above illustrations show the difference between a brain with normal activity (left) and a brain that has been atrophied because of Alzheimer's (right).

Sources: "Understanding Stem Cells," The National Academies, October 2006. http://dels.nas.edu; "The Changing Brain in Alzheimer's Disease," National Institute on Aging, August 29, 2006. www.nia.nih.gov.

- According to the **National Kidney Foundation, 17 people** die every day while waiting for a transplant of a vital organ such as a heart, kidney, pancreas, lung, or bone marrow.

Stem Cell Treatment and Cancer Survival (1960–2003)

Years ago, people who were diagnosed with myeloma (cancer of the bone marrow), Hodgkin's and non-Hodgkin's lymphoma (cancer of the immune system), and leukemia (cancer of the blood), were almost certainly doomed to die. Today, the survival rate for these cancers has markedly improved due in part to treatments from bone marrow and umbilical cord stem cells.

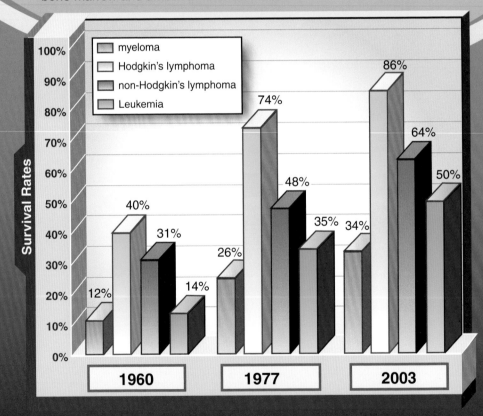

Source: "Facts 2007–2008," Leukemia and Lymphoma Society, June 2007. www.leukemia-lymphoma.org.

- In a clinical trial announced in 2007, **15 patients** with **type 1 diabetes** were treated with transfusions of stem cells drawn from their own blood and were able to stop taking insulin injections because their bodies began producing the hormone naturally.

Stem Cell Research and Organ Transplants

One of the reasons scientists are so excited about stem cell research is the potential of growing human organs in the laboratory. This has already been accomplished in several experiments, and if the technique is perfected, it is possible that organs grown from stem cells could greatly increase the supply of organs and tissues needed for transplantation— and could save thousands of lives every year. Currently there are significant shortages of all types of organs; as a result, many people die while waiting for transplants. The following chart shows the breakdown of the transplants performed versus the number of patients who need them.

Organ	Number of Transplants in 2006	Number of Patients on Waiting List
Kidney	17,092	70,870
Liver	6,650	16,946
Heart	2,192	2,847
Lung	1,405	2,817
Kidney/Pancreas	924	2,375
Pancreas	462	1,733
Intestine	175	229
Heart/Lung	31	121

Source: "25 Facts About Organ Donation and Transplantation," National Kidney Foundation, 2008. www.kidney.org.

Can the Stem Cell Debate Be Resolved?

> **Science works best when scientists can pursue all avenues of research. If the cure for Parkinson's disease or juvenile diabetes lay behind one of four doors, wouldn't you want the option to open all four doors at once instead of one door?**
>
> —Story Landis, quoted in Rick Weiss, "NIH Official Says Stem Cell Policy Is Delaying Cures."

> **The debate over embryonic stem cell research will never prove simple. Congress isn't always the best forum to hash out complicated bioethical issues. But it appears inevitable that we will confront these questions time and again as science advances.**
>
> —Bill Frist, "Meeting Stem Cells' Promise—Ethically."

These days, anyone who scans articles on the Internet, watches television news, or peruses the newspaper, undoubtedly hears or reads something about stem cells—and soon realizes that the issue is mired in controversy. Stem cell research has divided political parties, religious groups, and medical and research organizations, because beliefs are often so fundamentally different. Most people agree on the importance of stem cells and their potential for improving human health and prolonging lives. The crux of the debate is typically over the kinds of stem cells that should be used in research and whether methods of obtaining them are acceptable or unacceptable. As the controversy has continued to accelerate over the years, it has become increasingly contentious, which means it is not likely to disappear anytime in the near future.

A Long, Tedious Process

Even if the stem cell debate were resolved today and scientists throughout the world focused on nothing but stem cell research around the clock, it would still be years before treatments were available to benefit large numbers of patients. In the United States all new medical procedures, drugs, vaccinations, and treatments (including tissue transplants and stem cell therapies) must go through rigorous, time-consuming processes before they can be used on humans. First they must be proven safe and effective in numerous animal tests. If a treatment passes those tests, the FDA evaluates the data and decides if human clinical trials are in order. These trials are tightly regulated and generally happen in three or more phases. According to Christopher Thomas Scott, the first phase, which is to determine the safety and possible side effects of the treatment, involves only a few dozen subjects. The second phase determines the effectiveness of the treatment in several hundred patients, while the third phase (and possibly subsequent phases for continued testing) focuses on evaluating the treatment's significance and effectiveness in hundreds or thousands of patients. After all these steps have been completed and the FDA gives its approval, the treatment can be marketed to the public. Scott explains the complexity and expense of such a process: "Developing a new therapy goes slowly and is *terribly* expensive—discovering, testing, and manufac-

> Even if the stem cell debate were resolved today, and scientists throughout the world focused on nothing but stem cell research around the clock, it would still be years before treatments were available to benefit large numbers of patients.

turing one new drug can take between 10 and 15 years and cost nearly a billion dollars."[38]

By far, embryonic stem cell research faces the biggest hurdles because it is still in its infancy. Due to safety concerns, testing is limited to animals, and no human clinical trials have been approved. People who oppose the research are quick to point that out, saying that all the supposed benefits of embryonic stem cells are based on theories rather than actual proof. As science writer Michael Fumento explains:

> If you or a loved one is currently ill or planning to be so anytime in the near future, don't bother looking to embryonic stem cell (ESC) research to help. . . . At this point, all that ESCs hold is promise. They are used in no treatments, cures, or human clinical trials. They *are* used in raising false hopes and hence money. . . . When will the ESC promise pay off? When can we expect something more from them than arcane articles in medical journals? . . . You know, like, well, actually making sick people better?[39]

Fumento and others who share his viewpoint say that the greatest potential is with adult stem cells and other promising sources such as stem cells in amniotic fluid, and these are the areas that should be aggressively pursued.

Stem Cells and Politics

To say that stem cell research is a political issue would be a gross understatement—it is embroiled in political controversy, from arguments for and against embryonic stem cells to the debate over the ethics of cloning. It is not uncommon for politicians to bring up stem cells whenever they talk about today's most pressing issues, and they are often quite outspoken about their viewpoints. According to Sam Berger of the Center for American Progress, these politicians are out of touch with their constituents and oblivious to what the American people really want. He explains: "An overwhelming number of Americans support stem cell research, which politicians would know if they bothered to actually listen to them. It is time to abandon the old stem cell debate, fueled by a small but vocal minority, and begin focusing on the debate Americans want to have about how this research should be conducted."[40]

Stem cell research has been a subject of close scrutiny and debate for many years, but it rose to the forefront of the political arena in 2001. In August of that year, George W. Bush gave a televised address about stem cell funding, saying that his administration had crafted a policy that would fund human embryonic stem cell research. This had never happened in the past. Other presidents had discussed such funding, but Bush was the first to actually approve it. There was a caveat, however; he made it clear that the funds could be used only for research on existing embryonic stem cell lines. No federal funds would be granted for use in the destruction of human embryos, even those left over in fertility clinics that would likely be destroyed anyway. In 2006 and 2007 Bush used his veto power to reject proposed legislation that would expand federal funding to include newly developed stem cell lines, and Congress was not able to override the vetoes.

> To say that stem cell research is a political issue would be a gross understatement—it is embroiled in political controversy, from arguments for and against embryonic stem cells to the debate over the ethics of cloning.

Bush has been widely criticized for his refusal to fund new embryonic stem cell research. He has also been accused of banning the research, which is erroneous because he did not. In fact, embryonic stem cell research is flourishing in the United States, but most of it is financed by private or state funding rather than federal funds. In 2004 New Jersey became the first state to appropriate money for stem cell research by designating $10 million to be spread over 10 years. In November 2004 California voters approved Proposition 71, which allowed for the creation of a major stem cell research organization funded by $3 billion in state funds over 10 years. Other states have followed suit: Connecticut approved $100 million in state funding for embryonic stem cell research, Illinois designated $10 million, and New York designated $600 million.

Are Stem Cell Laws Too Restrictive?

As promising as stem cell therapy is, the development of human treatments is not progressing as fast as many people would like. One major reason is the law: In the United States the use of stem cells for human treatments is strictly controlled by the FDA. Embryonic stem cells are prohibited from being used in human clinical trials until they are proven to be safe. Umbilical cord blood is permissible only for treating certain diseases such as leukemia and anemia. Even the use of stem cells from a patient's own bone marrow is restricted by the FDA, and other types of adult stem cell treatments are still limited to use in animal experiments and some human clinical trials.

In a desperate effort to find a cure, many people who suffer from diseases or injuries travel to other countries where stem cell treatment laws are less restrictive. The Steenblock Institute is located in California but often refers patients to a medical facility in Mexico where umbilical cord stem cell treatments have been common for several years. According to David Steenblock and Anthony Payne, doctors and scientists in the United States commonly hold the belief that umbilical cord stem cells can only become red blood cells and certain immune system cells. Steenblock and Payne disagree, saying that "accumulating evidence indicates that umbilical cord stem cells can turn into a number of different cell types, benefiting neurological conditions such as cerebral palsy, early to middle-state multiple sclerosis [MS], early state atrophic lateral sclerosis [Lou Gehrig's disease], and certain eye and blood vessel diseases and conditions."[41] Steenblock and Payne say that patients have been successfully treated in Mexico for MS, cerebral palsy, ALS, and brain injuries, among others.

India is another country with stem cell laws that are less restrictive than the United States. It is legal to practice experimental stem cell treatments in India on patients whose injuries or diseases are deemed permanent or incurable. During the summer of 2007, Colorado native Amanda Boxtel traveled to Delhi, India, for stem cell therapy. Boxtel had been confined to a wheelchair since 1992, when a skiing accident left her paralyzed. Over a 2-month period she underwent the experimental therapy, which she hoped would restore movement in her legs. She describes the procedure and its effects on her: "With each vial or syringe, they would give me over 50 million stem cells. A catheter would be inserted into my spinal cord, and I could feel the stem cells like liquid jelly bleeding into my lower limbs. I could feel everything coming to life, literally, and things did. It's as though the stem cells fired up the cells and nerves in my body. It was instantaneous."[42] Boxtel's continued improvement has proven to her that the therapy did indeed "fire up" the cells in her body. Prior to the surgery she could not move her legs at all. Afterward, she could wiggle her toes, was noticeably more flexible, and her back muscles were stronger around her spine. Another benefit was a significant reduction in the burning pain that she constantly felt in her legs. She also says that her energy level has markedly increased—and for the first time in more than 15 years, she is able to stand up with the help of leg braces.

Should Embryonic Stem Cell Research Be Phased Out?

Because of all the promising research with stem cells that do not come from embryos, some people are convinced that this should be the focus rather than embryonic stem cell research. They argue that millions of dollars in funding is being wasted on a type of research that has never proven to be effective in treating humans and may never live up to its expectations. James Sherley shares his views: "Despite similar misinformation to the contrary, adult stem cell research is a viable and vibrant path to new medical therapies. Even [calling this research] an alternative to embryonic stem cells misinforms the public. Why? Because embryonic stem cells provide no path at all."[43]

> " In a desperate effort to find a cure, many people who suffer from diseases or injuries travel to other countries where stem cell treatment laws are less restrictive [than in the United States]. "

Yet many other scientists are convinced that if stem cell research is ever going to reach its full potential, all avenues must be pursued. In 2007 after James A. Thomson and Shinya Yamanaka announced their revolutionary discoveries with ordinary skin cells, this was hailed as the answer to one of the world's most pressing ethical dilemmas. Opponents of embryonic stem cell research embraced

> **The public may . . . be misled by the media when research findings are incorrectly interpreted or reported prematurely.**

the findings, saying that the pursuit of human embryonic research was no longer needed. Numerous researchers, including Thomson, disagreed, saying that although the findings were promising, embryonic stem cell research was still crucial. "A new way to trick skin cells into acting like embryos changes both everything and nothing at all," says Thomson. "Being able to reprogram skin cells into multipurpose stem cells without harming embryos launches an exciting new line of research. It's important to remember, though, that we're at square one, uncertain at this early stage whether souped-up skin cells hold the same promise as their embryonic cousins do."[44]

Is the Public Being Misled About Stem Cell Research?

People often form strong opinions about stem cells and typically get their information from the media. Unfortunately, not everything that is written about stem cell research is factual, which makes it difficult for anyone to fully understand the issue. Media reports are often incomplete or based on limited facts. One example is the repeated reference in news articles to the hundreds of thousands of embryos that are frozen in fertility clinics and available for research. While it is true that a likely 400,000 or more embryos are currently being preserved, that does not mean that they are "available for research." These embryos still belong to parents who, in many cases, have not decided what to do with them. No one knows for sure how many parents may be willing to donate embryos, and to say that they are readily available for research is deceptive.

The public may also be misled by the media when research findings are incorrectly interpreted or reported prematurely. According to Gareth Cook, people on all sides of the stem cell issue have distorted facts, and often this is because stem cell research is complex and not well understood. One example is research that was conducted in 1998 by Catherine Verfaille, a scientist at the University of Minnesota. In studying adult stem cells from bone marrow, Verfaille and her research team discovered an unexpected type of stem cell: an adult stem cell that appeared to have as much potential as embryonic stem cells, including the ability to become any cell in the body. When the research was announced in 2002, it caused a sensation in the scientific world. It was heralded by the media, touted by right-to-life advocates, gushed over in editorials, and praised by opponents of embryonic stem cell research. But all the excitement and media hype were premature. When other reputable researchers could not replicate the work, its true worth became doubtful. Even Verfaille herself expressed frustration with the politicization of the issue. "My research is being misused depending on the point someone wants to get across," she says. "They have put words in my mouth."[45]

A Never-Ending Debate?

Stem cell research has been discussed and debated for more than a decade, and that will undoubtedly continue in the years to come. There are many facets of the issue that need to be ironed out before any sort of a consensus can be reached on what should be legal, what should be funded, what should end, and what should continue. As time goes by and diseases and injuries continue to claim the lives of millions of people, politicians and other decision makers will likely be pressured by the public to resolve their differences and push stem cell research ahead. In spite of the controversy, however, most scientists are convinced that stem cells have the ability to change the future of human health forever.

Can the Stem Cell Debate Be Resolved?

❝There are camps for adult stem cells and embryonic stem cells. But these camps only exist in the political arena. There is no disagreement among scientists over the need to aggressively pursue both in order to solve important medical problems.❞

—Douglas Melton, quoted in Nancy Gibbs, "Stem Cells: The Hope and the Hype," *Time*, August 7, 2006.

Melton is codirector of the Harvard Stem Cell Institute.

❝Three-quarters of the U.S. public supports stem cell research that does not involve human embryos.❞

—Virginia Commonwealth University, "Widespread Support for Nonembryonic Stem Cell Research, VCU Life Sciences Survey Shows," news release, December 19, 2007. www.eurekalert.org.

Virginia Commonwealth University is the largest university in Virginia and is among the country's top research institutions.

Bracketed quotes indicate conflicting positions.

* Editor's Note: While the definition of a primary source can be narrowly or broadly defined, for the purposes of Compact Research, a primary source consists of: 1) results of original research presented by an organization or researcher; 2) eyewitness accounts of events, personal experience, or work experience; 3) first-person editorials offering pundits' opinions; 4) government officials presenting political plans and/or policies; 5) representatives of organizations presenting testimony or policy.

❝As often happens in science, stem cell research has raised as many new questions as it has answered, but the field is advancing. . . . The . . . hurdles are difficult but not insurmountable.❞

—Robert Lanza and Nadia Rosenthal, "The Stem Cell Challenge: What Hurdles Stand Between the Promise of Human Stem Cell Therapies and Real Treatments in the Clinic?" *Scientific American*, May 24, 2004.

Lanza and Rosenthal are leading stem cell researchers.

❝In this country, it is almost as if we would rather argue than find a solution. It would be so much better if we could find a way to produce these cells with a genuine social consensus behind them.❞

—William B. Hurlbut, quoted in Gareth Cook, "New Technique Eyed in Stem-Cell Debate," *Boston Globe*, November 21, 2004. www.boston.com.

Hurlbut is a physician and consulting professor at Stanford University's Neuroscience Institute.

❝President George W. Bush has banned all federal funding for research on human embryonic stem cells.❞

—Mira Oberman, "2007: Year of the Stem Cell," Discovery Channel, December 26, 2007. http://dsc.discovery.com.

Oberman is a journalist from Canada.

❝Contrary to the common myth, Bush never 'banned' stem-cell research, or even federal funding for it. Instead, he permitted such funding, for the first time, in a way that could help basic science advance while not encouraging the ongoing destruction of human embryos.❞

—*National Review*, "Stem-Cell Success," editorial, December 17, 2007.

National Review is a conservative public opinion magazine.

❝Resolution of the ethical and religious objections to stem cell research will doubtless take some time. If our society is to reach a consensus of sorts on this issue, a substantial growth in public understanding will be required.❞

—Donald Kennedy, quoted in Christopher Thomas Scott, *Stem Cell Now*. New York: Penguin, 2006.

Kennedy is editor in chief of *Science*, the American Association for the Advancement of Science's weekly journal.

❝Somewhere between the flat-earthers who would gladly stop progress and the swashbucklers who disdain limits are people who approve of stem-cell research in general but get uneasy as we approach the ethical frontiers.❞

—Nancy Gibbs, "Stem Cells: The Hope and the Hype," *Time*, August 7, 2006.

Gibbs is an editor at large for *Time* magazine.

❝This debate is one of the most profound ethical issues of all times. It has moral, religious, legal, and ethical overtones.❞

—Ron Paul, "Ron Paul's Speeches and Statements," July 31, 2001. www.house.gov.

Paul is a U.S. congressman representing a district of Texas.

❝Politicians don't want to enter this quagmire of ethics and science if they don't have to. There's no real middle ground—no compromise to be had.❞

—Patrick Kelly, quoted in Christine Vestal, "Embryonic Stem Cell Research Divides," Stateline.org, June 21, 2007. www.stateline.org.

Kelly is vice president for government affairs at the Biotechnology Industry Organization in Washington, D.C.

66 Discomfort with the notion of extracting stem cells from embryos is understandable. But many of the life-changing medical advances of recent history, including heart transplantation, have provoked discomfort. Struggling with bioethical questions remains a critical step in any scientific advancement. 99

—Alan I. Leshner and James A. Thomson, "Standing in the Way of Stem Cell Research," *Washington Post*, December 3, 2007. www.washingtonpost.com.

Leshner is chief executive of the American Association for the Advancement of Science, and Thomson is an embryologist and professor of anatomy at the University of Wisconsin School of Medicine and Public Health.

66 With continued support for non-destructive alternatives, new developments will continue to unfold in this field in the years to come, holding the potential for innovative progress toward new medical cures, while at the same time upholding human dignity and the sanctity of innocent life. 99

—Domestic Policy Council, "Advancing Stem Cell Science Without Destroying Human Life," White House, January 9, 2007. www.whitehouse.gov.

The Domestic Policy Council offers policy advice to the president of the United States on such issues as education, health, justice, welfare, environment, and veterans affairs.

Facts and Illustrations

Can the Stem Cell Debate Be Resolved?

- In 2006 Bush issued the **first veto of his presidency** by rejecting the Stem Cell Research Enhancement Act of 2005, which would have expanded funding for stem cell research to include the use of new additional embryos.

- In 2007 Bush vetoed the **Stem Cell Enhancement Act of 2007.**

- A December 2007 poll conducted by Virginia Commonwealth University showed that **46 percent** of respondents believed government regulation of stem cell research is necessary to protect the public, while **39 percent** said government regulation did more harm than good.

- A **May 2006 poll** by Opinion Research Corporation showed that **70 percent** of respondents favored expanded funding for embryonic stem cell research.

- In an August 2006 poll conducted by Princeton Survey Research Associates International, when respondents were asked their opinions of President Bush's handling of federal funding for stem cell research, **31 percent** approved and **52 percent** disapproved.

- The Stem Cell Resource, one of the **first privately funded**, nonprofit embryo banks in the United States, was founded in 2003 by fertility doctor David Smotrich, who **invested nearly $300,000** of his own money to start the bank.

Stem Cell Regulation Throughout the World

The United States and several other countries have laws in place that strictly regulate stem cell research as well as any treatments that may result from it. That is not the case everywhere in the world, however. Some countries have permissive laws, while others have no stem cell regulation at all.

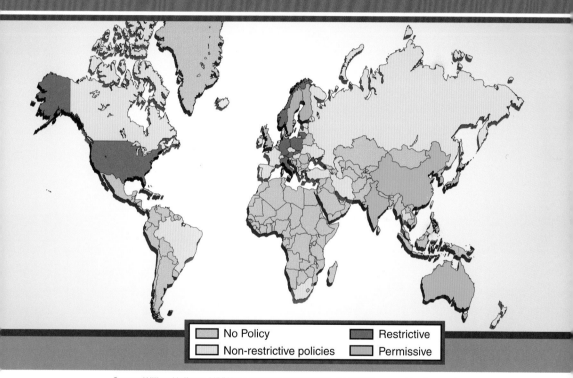

No Policy
Non-restrictive policies
Restrictive
Permissive

Source: William Hoffman, MBBNet, University of Minnesota, April 2007. www.mbbnet.umn.edu.

- In a May 2007 Gallup poll, **22 percent** of participants said that there should be no restrictions on government funding of stem cell research, up from **11 percent** in a 2005 poll.

- In a January 2007 CBS News poll, **43 percent** of participants favored the increase of federal spending on medical research using embryonic stem cells, up from **39 percent** in a 2006 poll.

Federally Funded Stem Cell Research

On August 9, 2001, President George W. Bush announced that he would approve federal funding for research on the embryonic stem cell lines already in existence. Since 2003, the National Institutes of Health (NIH) has provided more than $3.5 billion for stem cell research, embryonic as well as other types.

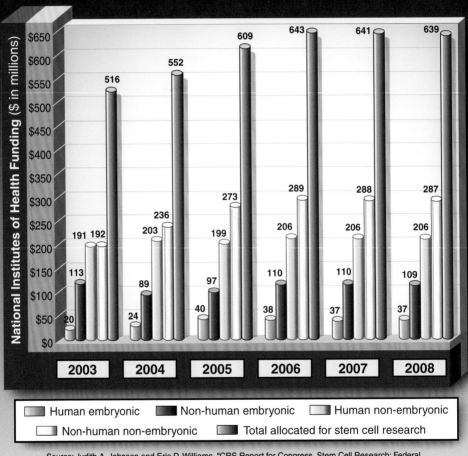

Source: Judith A. Johnson and Eric D. Williams, "CRS Report for Congress, Stem Cell Research: Federal Research Funding and Oversight," Congressional Research Service, April 18, 2007. http://fas.org.

- In April 2008 researchers at Yale School of Medicine identified, characterized, and **cloned ovarian cancer stem cells**, and found that the cells may be the source of ovarian cancer's recurrence and resistance to chemotherapy.

State-Funded Stem Cell Research

Because federal funding is restrictive and not available to researchers who create new embryonic stem cell lines, some states have set up their own funding entities, with monies allocated from state government and private sources.

New Jersey
In 2004 New Jersey became the first state to support stem cell research allocating $10 million to be distributed over 10 years to laboratories. Since then, lawmakers have appropriated another $15 million for grants and $9.5 million to cover administrative costs of the program. In 2007 New Jersey's governor signed legislation for another $270 million to build and equip 5 stem cell and biomedical research facilities.

California
In 2004 California voters approved Proposition 71, a funding program that would allocate $3 billion over 10 years. In June 2007, the California Institute of Regenerative Medicine approved grants of $50 million for stem cell research at 17 academic and nonprofit institutions.

Connecticut
Connecticut legislation passed in 2005 provided $100 million in state funding over 10 years for embryonic stem cell research.

Illinois
In 2005 the governor of Illinois directed the public health department in to grant $10 million to stem cell projects over 10 years and added $5 million more to the fund in July 2006. In August 2006 the Illinois Regenerative Medicine Institute granted $5 million to 7 projects at Illinois public universities.

Maryland
In 2006 the governor or Maryland signed a measure appropriating $15 million in general funds for stem cell research to be distributed in 2007.

Wisconsin
The state of Wisconsin created a $750 million investment fund, including public and private money, to build a research facility where embryonic stem cell studies may be conducted.

New York
In 2007 New York legislators created the Empire State Stem Cell Trust to support research on stem cells from any source. A total of $600 million was allocated; $100 million was earmarked for 2007–2008.

Massachusetts
In January 2008 the governor of Massachusetts proposed $1 billion for research followed by $50 million per year for the next 10 years.

Sources: "Stem Cell Research," National Conference of State Legislatures, January 2008. www.ncsl.org; Christine Vestal, "States Take Sides on Stem Cell Research," StateLine.org, January 31, 2008. www.stateline.org.

Key People and Advocacy Groups

George W. Bush: Bush, the forty-third president of the United States, was the first U.S. president to approve federal funding for embryonic stem cell research, as long as it was limited to stem cell lines that existed prior to August 2001 and did not involve the destruction of new human embryos.

Michael J. Fox: Fox, a well-known television and film actor who suffers from Parkinson's disease, founded the Michael J. Fox Foundation for Parkinson's Research and is a spokesperson on behalf of stem cell research.

Orrin Hatch: Hatch is a Republican U.S. senator and staunch right-to-life advocate who has been very outspoken about his support of embryonic stem cell research.

Hwang Woo-suk: A Korean researcher, Hwang was hailed throughout the world for being the first to create human embryonic stem cell lines from cloned embryos but was later disgraced after his claims turned out to be fraudulent.

International Society for Stem Cell Research (ISSCR): The ISSCR has been instrumental in promoting the importance of stem cell research, as well as promoting professional and public education about stem cell research and its applications.

National Institutes of Health (NIH): NIH scientists search for ways to improve human health as well as investigate the causes, treatments, and possible cures for diseases, including the use of stem cells.

Nancy Reagan: After her husband, the late Ronald Reagan, was stricken with Alzheimer's disease, Nancy Reagan became an outspoken advocate of all kinds of stem cell research.

Christopher Reeve: After a horseback-riding accident left him a quadriplegic in 1995, Reeve became one of America's most outspoken advocates on behalf of embryonic stem cell research; along with his wife, Dana, Reeve started the Christopher and Dana Reeve Foundation to aid victims of spinal cord injury.

E. Donnall Thomas: A Nobel Prize–winning physician, Thomas is credited with performing the world's first bone marrow transplant on a patient who suffered from leukemia.

James A. Thomson: Thomson is world-renowned as the first scientist to isolate human embryonic stem cells in 1998; in 2007 he again garnered worldwide fame as one of the scientists who successfully reprogrammed normal human skin cells to become stem cells with all the versatility and pluripotency of embryonic stem cells.

Shinya Yamanaka: A Japanese researcher, Yamanaka, independently of James A. Thomson, successfully reprogrammed normal human skin cells to become stem cells with all the versatility and pluripotency of embryonic stem cells.

Chronology

1839
German scientist Theodor Schwann theorizes that cells are the basic structural unit of all animals.

1969
E. Donnall Thomas performs the world's first bone marrow transplant on a patient whose donor was not a twin.

1963
In experiments with mice, Canadian researchers Ernest McCulloch and James Till find that stem cells have the ability to differentiate into a wide variety of new blood cells.

1981
Scientists from the United States and United Kingdom become the first to isolate and culture embryonic stem cells from mice. Researcher Gail R. Martin coins the term "embryonic stem cell."

1800   1950   1960   1970   1980   1990

1956
E. Donnall Thomas performs the world's first bone marrow transplant in New York, in which a patient with leukemia is cured by stem cells from his twin.

1978
Stem cells are discovered in umbilical cord blood and named hematopoietic stem cells.

Louise Joy Brown, a baby conceived through in vitro artificial insemination, is born in England and becomes known as the world's first "test tube baby."

1968
Robert A. Good performs the first bone marrow transplant on an infant with an inherited immune deficiency disorder, and the patient is cured.

British researchers Robert Edwards and Barry Bavister successfully fertilize a human egg with human sperm in a petri dish, which paves the way toward in vitro fertilization.

1988
The first umbilical cord blood transplant is used to treat and cure a young Parisian boy who was born with the potentially fatal blood disease Fanconi anemia.

2008

Scientists from McEwen Centre for Regenerative Medicine in Toronto, Canada, announce that they have created human master heart cells, able to transform into all the different cells that make up a beating heart, from embryonic stem cells. When implanted into mice, the cells improve the creatures' damaged hearts without forming teratomas.

1990

E. Donnall Thomas is awarded the Nobel Prize in Medicine for his work on bone marrow transplants.

1995

James A. Thomson creates the first embryonic stem cell line derived from monkeys.

2005

Korean researcher Hwang Woo-suk announces that he has developed 11 embryonic stem cell lines from cloned embryos. His claims are later proven to be fraudulent.

Senate Majority Leader Bill Frist, a Republican from Tennessee, announces his support of legislation that would loosen federal restrictions on embryonic stem cell research.

1990   **1995**   **2000**   **2005**

1998

Thomson leads a team of researchers at the University of Wisconsin at Madison to isolate and grow the first human embryonic stem cells.

2001

George W. Bush becomes the first U.S. president to approve federal funding for embryonic stem cell research, but limits the funding to stem cell lines that already exist.

2006

In his first presidential veto, Bush rejects the Stem Cell Enhancement Act, which would have expanded federal funding to cover new embryonic stem cell research.

2007

Anthony Atala leads a team of researchers from Wake Forest University School of Medicine to discover that stem cells found in amniotic fluid appear to have as much potential for pluripotency as embryonic stem cells.

Bush vetoes the Stem Cell Enhancement Act of 2007.

Researchers James A. Thomson of the United States and Shinya Yamanaka of Japan grow embryonic-like stem cells from ordinary human skin cells.

Related Organizations

American Association for the Advancement of Science (AAAS)

1200 New York Ave. NW

Washington, DC 20005

phone: (202) 326-6400 • fax: (202) 371-9526

e-mail: webmaster@aaas.org • Web site: www.aaas.org

The AAAS is an international organization that is dedicated to advancing science around the world and that strongly advocates stem cell research. Publications available through its Web site include the journal Science, EurekAlert! news service, and other scientific newsletters, books, and reports.

Americans for Cures Foundation

550 S. California Ave., Suite 330

Palo Alto, CA 94306

phone: (650) 812-9303 • fax: (650) 833-0105

e-mail: inform@americansforcures.org

Web site: www.americansforcures.org

Americans for Cures Foundation (previously known as the Alliance for Stem Cell Research) is dedicated to supporting stem cell advocates in the quest to expand research and find cures for chronic diseases and disabilities. Its Web site offers links to articles about stem cells, a Stem Cell Facts section, and a FAQs list related to stem cells.

Bedford Stem Cell Research Foundation

PO Box 1028

Bedford, MA 01730

phone: (617) 623-5670 • fax: (617) 623-9447

e-mail: info@bedfordresearch.org • Web site: www.bedfordresearch.org

Bedford Stem Cell Research Foundation is a biomedical organization whose focus is conducting stem cell and related research for diseases and disorders that currently have no effective treatment methods or cures. Its

Web site features a monthly newsletter, stem cell FAQs, current research information, and video clips of stem cells.

Biotechnology Industry Organization (BIO)

1201 Maryland Ave. SW, Suite 900

Washington, DC 20024

phone: (202) 962-9200 • fax: (202) 488-6301

e-mail: info@bio.org • Web site: www.bio.org

BIO is the world's largest biotechnology organization and a strong advocate of stem cell research. It provides advocacy, business development, and communications services for its membership, which is composed of a wide variety of organizations involved in research and development. The BIO Web site includes research articles, speeches and publications, state by state initiatives, and news releases.

Centers for Disease Control and Prevention (CDC)

1600 Clifton Rd.

Atlanta, GA 30333

phone: (404) 639-3534 or toll-free (800) 311-3435

fax: (800) 553-6323

e-mail: inquiry@cdc.gov • Web site: www.cdc.gov

The CDC, which is part of the U.S. Department of Health and Human Services, seeks to promote health and quality of life by controlling disease, injury, and disability. Its Web site features journals and other publications, an image library, statistical information, and links to many articles on stem cell research.

Coalition for the Advancement of Medical Research (CAMR)

2021 K St. NW, Suite 305

Washington, DC 20006

phone: (202) 725-0339

e-mail: camresearch@yahoo.com • Web site: www.camradvocacy.org

CAMR, which is composed of patient organizations, universities, and scientific societies, is dedicated to the advancement of stem cell research. Featured on the organization's Web site are news articles, public poll results, letters to the editor of various news publications, and press releases.

Do No Harm: The Coalition of Americans for Research Ethics

1100 H St. NW, Suite 700

Washington, DC 20005

phone: (202) 347-6840 • fax: (202) 347-6849

e-mail: media@stemcellresearch.org

Web site: www.stemcellresearch.org

Founded in 1999, Do No Harm is an organization devoted to educating the public about the importance of stem cell research, while at the same time believing that the destruction of human embryos is unethical and unnecessary for medical progress. Its Web site features links to newspaper articles, press releases, commentary, political testimony, and the *Stem Cell Report* online journal.

Genetics Policy Institute (GPI)

11924 Forest Hill Blvd., Suite 22

Wellington, FL 33414-6258

phone: (888) 238-1423 • fax: (561) 791-3889

Web site: www.genpol.org

GPI, which says it is the catalyst of the "pro-cures movement," seeks to educate the public, key decision makers, and the media about critical issues related to stem cell research. Its Web site's "News Room" features numerous stem cell news articles, editorials, and press releases, and more information is available in the site's "Pro-Cures" section.

Harvard Stem Cell Institute (HSCI)

42 Church St.

Cambridge, MA 02138

phone: (617) 496-4050

e-mail: hsci@harvard.edu • Web site: www.hsci.harvard.edu

HSCI, a Harvard University research organization, is committed to exploring both embryonic and adult stem cell research in an effort to advance the progress of stem cells and find new treatments for Parkinson's and other debilitating diseases. Its Web site offers the online publication *Stem Cell Lines* as well as monthly research newsletters, scientific overviews, and links to numerous articles about stem cell research.

International Society for Stem Cell Research (ISSCR)

111 Deer Lake Rd., Suite 100

Deerfield, IL 60015

phone: (847) 509-1944 • fax: (847) 480-9282

e-mail: isscr@isscr.org • Web site: www.isscr.org

The ISSCR seeks to encourage and promote the importance of stem cell research as well as professional and public education about stem cell research and application. Its Web site provides an online newsletter, the *Pulse*, as well as scientific literature about stem cells, resources on ethical issues, information on stem cell lines, and links to other sites of interest.

The National Academies

500 Fifth St. NW

Washington, DC 20001

phone: (202) 334-3313 • fax: (202) 334-2451

e-mail: (form available on Web site)

Web site: www.nationalacademies.org

The National Academies are composed of the National Academy of Sciences, National Academy of Engineering, Institute of Medicine, and National Research Council. The organization serves as an adviser to the federal government and the public on issues related to science, engineering, and medicine. Various stem cell publications are available on its Web site, including news releases, brochures, an e-newsletter, and the comprehensive booklet *Understanding Stem Cells*.

National Institutes of Health (NIH)

9000 Rockville Pike

Bethesda, MD 20892

phone: (301) 496-4000

e-mail: nihinfo@od.nih.gov • Web site: www.nih.gov

NIH, the leading medical research organization in the United States, is the primary federal agency responsible for conducting and supporting medical research. NIH scientists search for ways to improve human health as well as investigate the causes, treatments, and possible cures for diseases. Its Web site's Stem Cell Information section features a wealth of facts about stem cells, including "Stem Cell Basics," ethical issues, scientific literature, the NIH Stem Cells Registry, and U.S. policies on stem cell research.

National Organization for Rare Disorders (NORD)

55 Kenosia Ave.

PO Box 1968

Danbury, CT 06813-1968

phone: (203) 744-0100; toll-free: (800) 999-6673 (voicemail only)

fax: (203) 798-2291

e-mail: orphan@rarediseases.org • Web site: www.rarediseases.org

NORD is committed to the identification, treatment, and cure of rare disorders (known as "orphan" diseases) through programs of education, advocacy, research (including with stem cells), and service. The Web site features a database of rare diseases, news articles, speeches and testimonies, and position papers.

National Right to Life Committee (NRLC)

512 10th St. NW

Washington, DC 20004

phone: (202) 626-8800 • fax: (202) 347-3668

e-mail: nrlc@nrlc.org • Web site: www.nrlc.org

NRLC is a pro-life organization that describes its mission as "to restore legal protection to innocent human life." Although NRLC's primary interest has been the abortion debate, it is also concerned with medical ethics issues, including opposition to embryonic stem cell research. The Web site features editorials, a daily *Today's News and Views* online newsletter, and stem cell research materials.

For Further Research

Books

Michael Bellomo, *The Stem Cell Divide: The Facts, the Fiction, and the Fear Driving the Greatest Scientific, Political and Religious Debate of Our Time*. New York: American Management Association, 2006.

Cynthia B. Cohen, *Renewing the Stuff of Life: Stem Cells, Ethics, and Public Policy*. New York: Oxford University Press, 2007.

Cynthia Fox, *Cell of Cells: The Global Race to Capture and Control the Stem Cell*. New York: Norton, 2007.

Leo Furcht and William Hoffman, *The Stem Cell Dilemma*. New York: Arcade, 2008.

Eve Herold, *Stem Cell Wars: Inside Stories from the Frontlines*. New York: Palgrave Macmillan, 2006.

Suzanne Holland, Karen Lebacqz, and Laurie Zoloth, eds., *The Human Embryonic Stem Cell Debate: Science, Ethics, and Public Policy*. Cambridge, MA: MIT Press, 2001.

Robert Lanza, E. Donnall Thomas, James Thomson, and Roger Pedersen, *Essentials of Stem Cell Biology*. Boston: Elsevier/Academic, 2006.

Kristen Renwick Monroe, Ronald B. Miller, and Jerome S. Tobis, *Fundamentals of the Stem Cell Debate: The Scientific, Religious, Ethical, and Political Issues*. Berkeley and Los Angeles: University of California Press, 2008.

David E. Newton, *Stem Cell Research*. New York: Facts On File, 2007.

Christopher Thomas Scott, *Stem Cell Now*. New York: Penguin, 2006.

David A. Steenblock and Anthony G. Payne, *Umbilical-Cord Stem-Cell Therapy: The Gift of Healing from Healthy Newborns*. Laguna Beach, CA: Basic Health, 2006.

Brent Waters and Ronald Cole-Turner, *God and the Embryo: Religious Voices on Stem Cells and Cloning*. Washington, DC: Georgetown University Press, 2003.

Periodicals

Patrick Barry, "Hold the Embryos: Genes Turn Skin into Stem Cells," *Science News*, November 24, 2007.

Sharon Begley, "Reality Check on an Embryonic Debate," *Newsweek*, December 3, 2007.

Mary Carmichael, "Stem Cells Are Where It's At," *Newsweek*, December 11, 2006.

John W. Donohue, "The Stem Cell Debate: Why Is There an Irreconcilable Division Between Two Groups of Thoughtful and Sympathetic People?" *America*, November 13, 2006.

Emma Dorey, "Selling Snake Oil," *Chemistry and Industry*, December 4, 2006.

Nancy Gibbs, "Stem Cells: The Hope and the Hype," *Time*, August 7, 2006.

Bernadine Healy, "A Stem Cell Victory," *U.S. News & World Report*, January 14, 2008.

Matthew Herper and Robert Langreth, "Stem Cells: Billionaires vs. Bush," *Forbes*, September 4, 2006.

Michael Humphrey, "Advances Don't Quell Stem-Cell Debate," *National Catholic Reporter*, January 11, 2008.

Claudia Kalb and Debra Rosenberg, "Embryonic War; Scientists and Ethicists Put the Latest Stem-Cell 'Breakthrough' Under the Microscope," *Newsweek*, September 4, 2006.

Celeste Kennel-Shank, "No Time for Retreat: The Difficulty—and Necessity—of Finding a Middle Ground on Stem Cells," *Sojourners*, December 2007.

Michael Kinsley, "Why Science Can't Save the GOP," *Time*, December 10, 2007.

Deborah Kotz, "The Gift of a Cure (Stem Cell Banks)," *U.S. News & World Report*, May 21, 2007.

B.J. Lee, "Storm over Stem Cells," *Newsweek International*, January 9, 2006.

Nancy Frazier O'Brien, "Pro-Life Official Dismisses New Stem Cell Announcement as a Sham," *National Catholic Reporter*, December 15, 2006.

Brian O'Connell, "Stem Cell—Tough Sell on Wall Street?" *Biopharm International*, December 2006.

Mehmet C. Oz, "Breaking New Ground on Stem Cells: Embryonic Stem Cells Without Harming Embryos—New Research Opens Minds," *Saturday Evening Post*, March/April 2007.

Alice Park, "Stem Cells That Kill," *Time*, April 24, 2006.

Jamie Rosen, "Weird Science: Stem Cell Technology Makes Its Way to the Beauty Aisle," *W*, October 2007.

Wesley J. Smith, "Science and Spin; An 'Educational' Video on Stem-Cell Research Leaves Science in Disgrace," *Weekly Standard*, November 27, 2006.

Rosemary Tong, "Stem Cell Research and the Affirmation of Life," *Conscience*, Autumn 2006.

Karen Tumulty, "The Politics of Science," *Time*, August 7, 2006.

Arlene Weintraub, "What's Ethical and What Isn't? The Debate over Human Cells in Animals," *BusinessWeek*, January 16, 2006.

Rick Weiss, "Scientists See Potential in Amniotic Stem Cells," *Washington Post*, January 8, 2007.

Mortimer B. Zuckerman, "Some Hope on Stem Cells," *U.S. News & World Report*, September 11, 2006.

———, "Tiny Liver Grown from Umbilical Cord Stem Cells," *National Right to Life News*, November 2006.

Internet Sources

Charles Babington, "Stem Cell Bill Gets Bush's First Veto," *Washington Post*, July 20, 2006. www.washingtonpost.com/wp-dyn/content/article/2006/07/19/AR2006071900524.html.

Arthur Caplan, "The End of Stem Cell Research? Hardly," MSNBC, January 3, 2006. www.msnbc.msn.com/id/10683107.

Maureen L. Condic, "What We Know About Embryonic Stem Cells," *First Things: The Journal of Religion, Culture, and Public Life*, January 2007. www.firstthings.com/article.php3?id_article=5420.

Steven Edwards, "Thousands of Adult Stem Cell Deaths Show Urgency of Embryonic Research," *Wired*, April 11, 2007. www.wired.com/med tech/stemcells/commentary/spinalcolumn/2007/04/spinalcolumn_0411.

Ronald M. Green, "The Stem Cell Debate," *Life's Greatest Miracle*, *Nova*, PBS, November 20, 2001. www.pbs.org/wgbh/nova/miracle/stemcells.html.

Gina Kolata, "Man Who Helped Start Stem Cell War May End It," *New York Times*, November 22, 2007. www.nytimes.com/2007/11/22/science/22stem.html?_r=1&oref=slogin.

Robert Lanza and Nadia Rosenthal, "The Stem Cell Challenge," *Scientific American*, May 24, 2004. www.sciam.com/article.cfm?article ID=000DFA43-04B1-10AA-84B183414B7F0000&sc=I100322.

National Institutes of Health, "Stem Cell Information," December 30, 2006. http://stemcells.nih.gov/info/basics.

Nature Reports, "Stem Cells," 2008. www.nature.com/stemcells/index.html.

Michael J. Sandel, "Embryo Ethics," *Boston Globe*, April 8, 2007. www.boston.com/news/globe/ideas/articles/2007/04/08/embryo_ethics.

Stephanie Watson, "How Stem Cells Work," *How Stuff Works*. http://science.howstuffworks.com/stem-cell.htm.

Christine Vestal, "Embryonic Stem Cell Research Divides States," Stateline.org, June 21, 2007. www.stateline.org/live/details/story?contentId=218416.

Source Notes

Overview

1. Christopher Thomas Scott, *Stem Cell Now*. New York: Penguin, 2006, p. 27.
2. *Nature Reports: Stem Cells*, "What Are Stem Cells?" July 6, 2007. www.nature.com.
3. Gareth Cook, "From Adult Stem Cells Comes Debate," *Boston Globe*, November 1, 2004. www.boston.com.
4. Quoted in Scott, *Stem Cell Now*, p. xi.
5. Quoted in Colin Nickerson, "California Biotech Says It Cloned a Human Embryo, but No Stem Cells Produced," *Boston Globe*, January 17, 2008. www.boston.com.
6. Stem Cell Therapies, "What Are Stem Cells?" Steenblock Research Institute, 2004–2006. www.stemcelltherapies.org.
7. *Nature Reports: Stem Cells*, "What Are Stem Cells?"
8. Quoted in Amy Adams, "Stanford Q and A: Irving Weissman on the South Korea Stem Cell Controversy," news release, Stanford School of Medicine, December 20, 2005. http://med.stanford.edu.
9. Wesley J. Smith, "Cell Wars," *National Review*, June 8, 2004. www.nationalreview.com.
10. Quoted in Michael Cook, "Harvard's Stem Cell Misstep," *MercatorNet*, June 29, 2006. www.mercatornet.com.
11. Michael Kinsley, "Why Science Can't Save the GOP," *Time*, December 10, 2007, p. 36.
12. Quoted in Mira Oberman, "Stem Cell Breakthrough Is Like Turning Lead into Gold," *Brisbane Times*, December 24, 2007. www.brisbanetimes.com.au.
13. Maureen L. Condic, "What We Know About Embryonic Stem Cells," *First Things: The Journal of Religion, Culture, and Public Life*, January 2007. www.firstthings.com.
14. Quoted in Doug Trapp, "Bush Rejects Second Stem Cell Bill; Veto Override Is Unlikely," *AMNews*, July 9, 2007. www.ama-assn.org.

Is Stem Cell Research Necessary?

15. Quoted in Allan Madrid, "Prof Says Stem Cell Research Necessary, Beneficial," *Daily Northwestern*, January 13, 2005. www.dailynorthwestern.com.
16. Quoted in Tom Paulson, "Seattle Doc First to Use Stem Cells," *Seattle Post-Intelligencer*, September 28, 2007. http://seattlepi.nwsource.com.
17. Quoted in Scott, *Stem Cell Now*, p. 5.
18. Quoted in BBC News, "Cell Transplants 'Restore Sight,'" November 8, 2006. http://news.bbc.co.uk.
19. Quoted in Karen Kreeger, "New Source of Multipotent Adult Stem Cells Discovered in Human Hair Follicles," news release, University of Pennsylvania School of Medicine, July 12, 2006. www.uphs.upenn.edu.
20. Quoted in Karen Kaplan, "Stem Cells in Amniotic Fluid Show Promise," *Los Angeles Times*, January 8, 2007. www.latimes.com.
21. Scott, *Stem Cell Now*, p. 196.

Is Stem Cell Research Ethical?

22. George W. Bush, "The President Discusses Stem Cell Research Policy," White House news release, July 19, 2006. www.whitehouse.gov.
23. Scott, *Stem Cell Now*, p. 124.
24. Quoted in William J. Cromie, "Melton Derives New Stem Cell Lines," *Har-*

vard Gazette, March 4, 2004. www. hno.harvard.edu.

25. Quoted in CNN.com, "Research Foes Decry Embryo 'Slaughter,'" July 25, 2001. http://archives.cnn.com.

26. Michael J. Sandel, "Embryo Ethics," *Boston Globe*, April 8, 2007. www.boston.com.

27. Quoted in Brandon Keim, "Embryonic Stem Cells Created Without Harming Embryo, for Real This Time," *Wired*, January 10, 2008. www.wired.com.

28. Scott, *Stem Cell Now*, p. 124.

29. Charles Krauthammer, "Personal Statements," *Human Cloning and Human Dignity: An Ethical Inquiry*, July 2002. www.bioethics.gov.

30. Quoted in *BusinessWeek*, "Online Extra: Michael J. Fox's Take on Stem Cells," May 24, 2004. www.businessweek.com.

31. John F. Kilner, "Poor Prognosis for Preimplantation Genetic Diagnosis (PGD)?" Center for Bioethics and Human Dignity, August 6, 2004. www.cbhd.org.

32. Quoted in Gina Kolata, "Man Who Helped Start Stem Cell War May End It," *New York Times*, November 22, 2007. www.nytimes.com.

Are Stem Cells the Answer to Prolonged Human Life?

33. Anthony D. Ho, Wolfgang Wagner, and Ulrich Mahlknecht, "Stem Cells and Ageing," *EMBO Reports Science & Society*, vol. 6, 2005. www.nature.com.

34. Eve Herold, *Stem Cell Wars: Inside Stories from the Frontlines*. New York:

Palgrave Macmillan, 2006, p. 41.

35. Quoted in Lawrence K. Altman, "Team Creates Rat Heart Using Cells of Baby Rats," *New York Times*, January 14, 2008. www.nytimes.com.

36. Quoted in Scott, *Stem Cell Now*, p. 114.

37. National Institute on Aging, "The Changing Brain in Alzheimer's Disease," August 29, 2006. www.nia.nih.gov.

Can the Stem Cell Debate Be Resolved?

38. Scott, *Stem Cell Now*, p. 97.

39. Michael Fumento, "Adult Approaches: Will Embryonic Stem Cell Promise Ever Pay Off?" *American Spectator*, May 2007. www.fumento.com.

40. Sam Berger, "The Silent Stem Cell Majority," Center for American Progress, February 22, 2006. www.americanprogress.org.

41. David Steenblock and Anthony G. Payne, *Umbilical Cord Stem Cell Therapy*. Laguna Beach, CA: Basic Health, p. 37.

42. Quoted in Naomi Havlan, "Stem Cell Treatment Helps Boxtel Regain Strength," *Aspen Times*, August 23, 2007. www.aspentimes.com.

43. "James Sherley: No Path to Find Cure-All," *Australian*, October 12, 2006. www.theaustralian.news.com.au.

44. Alan I. Leshner and James A. Thomson, "Standing in the Way of Stem Cell Research," *Washington Post*, December 3, 2007. www.washingtonpost.com.

45. Quoted in Gareth Cook, "From Adult Stem Cells Comes Debate."

List of Illustrations

Index

About the Author

Peggy J. Parks holds a bachelor of science degree from Aquinas College in Grand Rapids, Michigan, where she graduated magna cum laude. She is an author who has written more than 60 nonfiction educational books for children and young adults and has self-published her own cookbook called *Welcome Home: Recipes, Memories, and Traditions from the Heart*. Parks lives in Muskegon, Michigan, a town that she says inspires her writing because of its location on the shores of Lake Michigan.